You are not necessarily "stuck" with your handwriting any more than you are "stuck" with personality defects or other flaws in inner make-up. You can change yourself by changing your handwriting!

Certain criteria in handwriting analysis can reveal your inner strengths and weaknesses—your handwriting is a mirror of you at this very moment.

Whether child or adult, entire lives have been changed for the better by this one tool—handwriting—an index to one's character, one's personality, even one's health.

Phyllis Harrison is also the author of
Pendulum, Radiesthesia, and You

HELPING YOUR HEALTH
THROUGH HANDWRITING

Second Edition

Completely revised and expanded

Foreword by Linda Clark

Phyllis Harrison

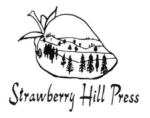

Strawberry Hill Press

Strawberry Hill Press
2594 15th Avenue
San Francisco, California 94127

Manufactured in the United States of America

Proofread by Kelly McCreight Ward

Wordprocessed by Joseph Lubow

Typeset by Cragmont/ExPress, Oakland, California

Printed by Edwards Brothers Incorporated, Ann Arbor, Michigan

Library of Congress Cataloging in Publication Data

Harrison, Phyllis, 1910—

    Helping your health through handwriting.

    Bibliography: p.
    1. Graphology. 2. Medicine. 3. Health.
I. Title.
BF905.M43H37 1985   155.2'82   85-10082
ISBN 0-89407-069-X (pbk.)

Dedication

This book is dedicated to several very dear and close friends who have helped me enormously in my work: Adolf Schoepe, president of Fluidmaster, Inc.; Laura Nickolsen; Don C. Matchan; Edward S. Hawkins of Richlore Foundation; Marian and Harold Van Patten; Linda Clark, the late noted nutrition reporter; and my nephew, Rhio H. Spray.

And to all those who so graciously allowed me to quote from their work in this volume.

FOREWORD

Handwriting, which some experts refer to as "brainwriting," can be an index to one's character, one's personality, even one's health. It is a mirror of *you* at this very moment, as proved in country after country—except America, where it is just beginning to catch on.

Any information on handwriting is liable to make you self-conscious about your handwriting, which you may consider poor, sloppy, or illegible. But making you self-conscious, or in some other way "putting you down," is not at all the purpose of this fine book. What you will learn, however, is that certain criteria in handwriting analysis can reveal your inner strengths and weaknesses, and have nothing to do with whether or not your writing is pretty.

Best of all, you are not necessarily "stuck" with your handwriting any more than you are "stuck" with personality defects or other flaws in inner make-up. You *can* change yourself by changing your handwriting! It has already been done by countless people, and this book tells *you* how to do it!

Such changes are not restricted to any particular age group—they are universal. Children's grades have improved and their personality faults have improved or disappeared; and exactly the same is true for adults of all ages. Whether child or adult, entire lives have been changed by this one tool alone. Believe me, there are exciting possibilities here.

Far out? Wierd? Not at all. Phyllis Harrison teaches college courses on handwriting and what it can do for you. She has testimonials galore to prove that it does work. She is a consultant to government, education, and business; several large corporations employ her to choose the right person for the right job (no more round pegs in square holes) on the basis of handwriting alone. And those fortunate workers, as well as the executives who hire them, marvel at the success of this method. Employers who did not accept her recommendations and did their own choosing often later regretted it.

Phyllis has helped many, many people spot health difficulties through their handwriting, and she, herself, is a vibrant example of what the method can accomplish. At one time she was ill and poorly adjusted; today she is energetic, healthy, and happy, with nary a hang-up. Her admirers are legion. A common remark by those who know her is: If Phyllis says it is so, you can depend on it. So, with Phyllis Harrison providing her research and knowledge about handwriting and what it can do, you can bank on it.

I recommend this book unreservedly.

—**Linda Clark**

Table of Contents

Graphology: What It Can Do for You

Do you ever have nagging doubts about yourself—and wonder why communication problems develop within your family, among co-workers, or with friends? Or are you the sort who wraps all the problems in a package labeled "They"? In traffic, at the office or plant, in the classroom, at church activities, at home—would everything be okay if "he" or "she" or "they" had acted differently?

Do some situations agitate you, mildly or to the point of panic, like going to work when you *know* the supervisor or boss will get uptight about something before the day is out? And when that happens, do you get upset too? Are there times when that old demon fear takes over, and the solar plexus knots up; or the adrenals get revved up and the heart goes doubletime, the face reddens, and the temperature rises? Oh, how it can split the skull wide open sometimes!

Do you have times when you think other people can do better work than you can? When a new assignment frightens you? Do you scare easily and let more aggressive people bluff you out of a decision, or into one that down deep you don't think is right?

Do you have a reservoir where you store **resentments**? It doesn't make too much difference who says or does it: it might be Friend Husband, The Wife, a Friend, or associates on the job. Of course, you don't always answer back—if it's the boss, hardly! And if you start snapping at "him" or "her" it may go on and on. And if someone hasn't said "I'm sorry" before bedtime, those inner mechanisms in the subconscious are still working, telling the adrenals the fight's still on, to keep cranking; telling the muscles to keep contorting, the hypothalamus to keep functioning, as if the enemy were going to get you if you don't get him first!

These may be adult situations—but perhaps you're a young adult, in high school or college, or still in the elementary grades—you *are* old enough to know that most "problems" are people-problems, right? *Things* don't really cause too many problems. When things get out of whack, you fix them or have a specialist do it. But maintaining easy, smooth relationships with other two-footed creatures—that's something else. You learned that before you could talk, really, though you weren't aware of it. But you did discover that when you wanted food, it helped to yell. Or when you wanted to go out and play, it helped to tease; and when you wanted a brightly packaged yum-yum in the market, maybe it helped to smile and tug at mom, or perhaps whine. You didn't know it then, but a well-known medical doctor, Dr. Thomas A. Harris, points out in his book *I'm O.K.-You're O.K.* that the first five years of life are the most crucial. We take on the attitudes our parents harbor and our human computer, the subconscious mind, stores them for future use. Too bad, isn't it, that the "bad" attitudes, the harmful ones that many years later can lead to physical illness and even death, are thus filed away?

You bet it's too bad! And that's what this book is all about: Searching out, discovering those elusive devils, and rooting them out of our thought-system, our belief-system, so we can function in harmony with our families and our everyday associates, and most importantly—*ourselves*.

When we get right with ourselves, other things start falling into place, miraculously some say, and the whole world changes. Get that? *The world changes*. And a sometimes-desolate, oftentimes hostile, rude, even brutal world is transformed into a pleasant, reasonably serene, often downright happy and carefree place!

Is this worth working toward? If your answer is yes, you're in the right pew with the right book. If, on the other hand, you have sold yourself the idea that you enjoy occasionally bringing out of the reservoir a resentment against so-and-so who slighted you, looked down on you, or did you dirt with the boss; or if you enjoy dredging up an ancient feeling of hurt toward someone in your family or an acquaintance, reliving the episode, restating the angry words that passed—this isn't the book for you.

What I'm trying to say is: An alcoholic or a chain-smoker doesn't put the habit on the skids until the moment arrives when he or she can say *I want to quit.* That's the starting point, the magic declaration that goes into the subconscious and chases the baddies out one by one—if the conviction and the determination for change is the dominant thought-command.

Our world is beautiful, can be beautiful, because its Maker decreed *freedom of choice.* Some things, like a political dictator, we may not free ourselves from. But anything that has to do with self, we can control. All we need to possess is knowledge, desire, and will. This book will provide the knowledge of how you, if you wish, can discover hidden gremlins in attitudes that actually dictate your behavior and how you respond to other human beings. And that response is the key to what can be happening in your "temple"—the only physical body you'll ever have on Planet Earth—or at least the only one you'll be able to recognize as yours. The secrets lie in your handwriting and they are not secrets to an analyst. As you learn the simple art of analysis, they will unfold to you.

Just as the scientist cannot tell us *why* invisible magnetic currents or waves carry sound and light and the weatherman can't tell us *why* some parts of the globe have four sharply different seasons, I cannot tell you *why* handwriting reflects your attitudes. But I *can* tell you *how* to read the signs; what they mean; and, most significantly, how you can eliminate those attitudes you know are destructive to your mental and physical health and replace them with constructive, blessed attitudes that bring inner peace, physical healing, spiritual serenity, and total harmony with the persons and events that we know as our world.

GRAPHOLOGY: A TOOL FOR UNDERSTANDING

Writing—a graphic expression—is the most direct means of evaluating character structure. The graphic expression is a "frozen gesture," a personality trail left behind by the writer. This graphic picture, when analyzed and interpreted by a trained analyst, yields information for a more complete understanding of the behavior of the writer—be it friend, client, loved one, or associate.

In the classroom milieu, graphology opens the door to an improved understanding and relationship between teacher and student. Through the writing of papers the student presents teacher with an up-to-the-minute image of how he's feeling, thinking, functioning. Any change in that "inner world" is unconsciously revealed, and the teacher gets the signal of worry, anxiety, happiness, loneliness. The sum of these signals, with others, alerts the teacher as to abilities and shortcomings that have made the student what he or she is at that moment in time.

Commonly believed a modern technique, graphology actually has roots nearly 2,000 years old. In A.D. 120, peculiarities in the handwriting of Emperor Octavius Augustus were noted by G. Suetonius Tranquillus in his book *Devita Caesarum*: "He does not hyphen the words and continue on to the following line, not even if this means cramming the letters, but simply squeezes them in and curves the end of the line downwards." And Justinian I, sixth-century ruler of the great Byzantine Empire, recorded in his memoirs that he was struck by the observation that one's handwriting changes with ill health and age.

The Chinese are reported as first to draw a correlation between personality and handwriting, a thousand years ago. But centuries passed before the first detailed work was authored in 1622 by Camillo Baldi, a professor for 59 years at the University of Bologna in Italy. The work was titled *Treating of How a Written Message May Reveal the Nature and Qualities of the Writer*. At 22, Baldi had received two degrees—Doctor of Philosophy, and Doctor of Medicine. His treatise *Of Gestures in General, and of the Voice* led to his study of handwriting as a projective technique.

Another 200 years passed before the French abbot Hippolyte Michon put graphology firmly on the map with the publication of an interpretive study of 10,000 handwriting samples. Today, as *The Wall Street Journal* writer David M. Elsner wrote (June 20, 1974), "Most graphologists agree on which quirks of handwriting reveal which personality quirks." Indeed, in the four centuries since Baldi's dissertation much, much more has been learned about the relationship between how you cross your *t*'s and dot your *i*'s, and how you respond to communication from others. Goethe, Lavater, Thomas Gainsborough, Walter Scott, Poe, Browning, Baudelaire, Kretzschmer, Bleuler, Jung, Einstein, were among those to make observations in published works and letters about handwriting.

Three German doctors and a scholar are credited with theoretical breakthroughs at the turn of the century. Physiologist

Wilhelm Preyer, and philosopher Ludwig Kages concluded that handwriting is not static, but rather is "dynamic, expressive movement, a result of fundamental function expressable in a variety of ways."

In 1895 Wilhelm Preyer termed handwriting "brainwriting," in that both the conscious and subconscious mind are imprinted in one's script. The phrase originated after he had observed a double amputee fluently produce his signature by holding a pen in the mouth. Dr. Preyer's colleagues expressed regret that "a scientist of merit should lose himself in the field of dangerous sciences, among which hypnosis and graphology belong."

Graphology has developed extensively in Europe — particularly Germany where practitioners are licensed by the government. Graphology courses are part of the curriculum in the German universities of Hamburg, Freiburg, Cologne, Mainz, Kiel, Munich, Berklin, Bonn, and Heidelberg. They require about three years for completion. Advanced courses have been taught at the Sorbonne in Paris, at Zurich, Berne, and Basel in Switzerland, and in Holland and Israel. And in 1966 Amsterdam hosted a session of the International Congress on Handwriting Psychology and Document Examination attended by 270 graphologists from 18 countries.

Business and industry are using graphology increasingly in personnel selection, and, of course, it is an accepted technique in criminal work. *Handwriting Analysis in Business* by N. Currer-Briggs *et al.*, reported in 1973 that about half the businesses in Germany use handwriting analysis in personnel placement; about two-thirds of Dutch firms rely on it as one means of psychological projection testing; and somewhat fewer businesses in France utilize it. The number of firms in the United States employing handwriting analysis to screen job applications and assist employees with work problems is estimated at more than 3,000 — a sharp rise from the beginning of the decade.

Edward J. Nouri, head of a New York agency of New England Mutual Life Insurance, says handwriting analysis tells him "more than a battery of psychological tests." Graphology is used by such corporations as IBM, Prudential Life, Boise Cascade, Stauffer Chemical, New York Life, Mutual of Omaha, Montgomery Ward, Spiegel Mail Order, and Manpower in this country, and I.G. Farben in Germany. At the Veterans Administration Hospital in

Minneapolis, MacBain Smith has used graphology for a quarter century. And San Francisco attorney Melvin Belli finds it useful in the preparation of lawsuits.

Use of graphology has lagged in this country, probably because of opposition within the medical and psychology communities. Scholars have spurned it, in the past, as "unscientific," "sheer guesswork," and "quackery." George K. Bennett, president of Psychological Corporation, New York, said some years back: "The evidence to date is insufficient to show that graphology has any value in predicting personality, character, intelligence, or any other trait. I wouldn't spend a plugged nickel on it." And to Alfred Kanfer's assertion that he could predict cancer through handwriting, the American Medical Association asserted: "There is absolutely no scientific validity to this guy's claims."

But recently there has been a literal explosion in the education in and use of graphology. Not only are colleges and universities teaching advanced classes in graphology, but students by the thousands have been graduating from classes taught in two-year colleges, adult programs in high schools, and private classes. Many of those same students have made contact with organized graphological societies for membership and further study. Seminars sponsored by those organized societies have proliferated and often provide the means whereby students begin to "network" with their peers.

In late 1980, at Carthage College, Kenosha, Wisconsin, there was a "historical first." It was a national conference, sponsored by the Council of Graphological Societies (COGS), to determine policies, standards, and criteria to fit the needs of all North American graphologists. The conference, for the first time in this country, adopted a code of ethics and policies acceptable to all schools of graphology.

While graphology has become fairly well standardized with the passage of time, practitioners in the United States still are neither licensed nor required to pass an accredited training course. However, the colleges and universities are showing more interest, probably due to the large number of graphologists who have graduated already from private schools and foundations. Many graphologists appear regularly on radio and T.V. throughout the United States.

Extensive research into handwriting is being conducted in Hungary, Germany, France, the Scandinavian countries, and in some parts of South America. And while academia in the United States still largely frowns on it, in European universities a requisite to practicing graphology is a degree in psychology. It is used in speech therapy, and to cope with reading problems; there is strong reason to suspect a link between handwriting "problems" and dyslexia.

PHYSICIANS ARE USING IT

Cyrus W. Loo, M.D., Hawaiian dermatologist, says he clears up some skin disorders by teaching patients to change their handwriting. A medical doctor at the University of Madrid uses graphotherapy to successfully treat psychological illnesses. And, Dr. Joaquin Alegret says, "I have case histories of purely organic cures on such conditions as throat disease, nervous diseases, and acute stomach troubles." The well-known psychologist-psychotherapist Herry O. Teltscher, Ph.D., notes in his book *Handwriting—Revelation of Self* that "Physicians are becoming more aware of handwriting as a means for detection of ailments not immediately apparent through medical checkups...and encouraging studies in the fields of psychosomatic medicine, malignant disease, and neuropsychiatry have been published in recent years. Mental and emotional disturbances have long been diagnosed through handwriting."

The late Alfred Kanfer, who fled Vienna during the Hitler years, was perhaps the first to utilize handwriting analysis to detect cancer. He spent the last years of his life at the Strang Clinic for Preventive Medicine, New York, examining handwriting for cancer signals, with 70%-80% accuracy.

Writing in the magazine *Psychic* (San Francisco, September, 1972), Robert W. Neubert related that: "In 1935 a young forged-document examiner for the Ministry of Justice in Vienna made a startling discovery. Alfred Kanfer observed what he maintains is a direct relationship between handwriting and cancer. He studied more than 35,000 signatures through the succeeding years, and today claims prediction accuracy of up to 97%.

"'The pen stroke of a normal person,' he says, 'when magnified under a microscope is smooth and continuous. But in cases where a cancer or precancerous condition is present, the magnified pen stroke looks like the segmented body of a caterpillar.... The pressure of pen and flow of ink on the paper has been interrupted by minute muscle twitches. There is a misfiring in the nerve messages to muscles—like the current in a faulty spark plug.

"'Changed behavior and changed movement may help indicate a developing physical disorder,' says Mr. Kanfer, noting however that handwriting alone does not give evidence of disease. Through a series of examples, he shows the script of persons before and after medical treatment. He shows that one individual with cancer of the bronchi had weak, pressureless, uneven loopings. Another person, several years after successful treatment for hyperthyroidism, wrote letters that appeared more self-assured, alert, and active. 'Handwriting is a direct and indirect record of the functions of the whole organism,' he says, 'It can be a valuable tool for both the physician and psychologist.'

"Mr. Kanfer says that as far as he knows 'there is no other accepted test that looks for hidden cancer in the whole body at once.' The American Cancer Society donated $10,000 to Mr. Kanfer in 1954 for a statistical study of the neuromuscular coordination effects of cancer. Terming results 'inconclusive,' the Society discontinued support.

"Daniel Miller, president and medical director of the Strang Clinic where Mr. Kanfer did much of his research, says he does not consider the Kanfer analysis a cancer test. Instead, he calls it 'a means of separating high-risk groups from low-risk groups on individuals.'

"Phil Moore, M.D., a surgeon in Porterville, California, who sometimes uses graphology in seeking to better understand the emotional problems of patients, says he is 'very reluctant to accept the idea that you can make a pathological or anatomical diagnosis from handwriting. At present it shouldn't be used as more than a guide to diagnosis.'

"The medical community," continues Mr. Neubert, "has held back from accepting Mr. Kanfer's invitation to 'sit down at the microscope and see for themselves.' Some graphologists say this is shortsighted, irresponsible, and immoral, especially since cancer still is a major unsolved disease."

Graphotherapist Raymond Trillat has been doing remarkable

work with disturbed children in Paris for many years.

The late Paul de Sainte Colombe writes in his *Grapho-therapeutics—Pen and Pencil Therapy* (Copyright, Mrs. Paul de Sainte Colombe, Hollywood, California) that "All types of abnormality (from slight mental and emotional disturbances to schizophrenia, paranoia, and sexual deviations) are discernible in handwriting, and this makes graphology a remarkable diagnostic tool, permitting the practitioner to go directly to the root of the patient's troubles...."

WHAT IS GRAPHOTHERAPY?

Now it's all very fine to be told your handwriting holds the secret to your "problems," but "So what?"—*unless you can do something about it*. Right? That's the beautiful part of this whole area of knowledge: It *is* available to you, where you are, *now*—at the precise moment you tell yourself, "I want to make some changes!"

And if you wonder how a seemingly simple process like doing handwriting exercises can help you regain mental/emotional/physical health—there's a physiological answer. Mr. de Sainte Colombe explains:

"Character sets the individual pattern of each handwriting, and is inseparable from it. Consequently, *a voluntary handwriting change*, once achieved, *produces a corresponding change of character*. How? The circuit established between brain and graphic gesture by the nervous system is two-way. Thus, the ability of the brain to influence the writing hand is reversible. Proof is demonstrated by a simple procedure most of us know from experience: That the act of setting down in writing information we want to remember, or memorize, implants it in the mind as nothing else can.

"Just as the subconscious mind affects handwriting, handwriting can be used to affect the subconscious mind. It can reinforce our neuroses, or eliminate them.

"The term 'graphotherapy' came into use around 1930, but the technique was introduced in November 1908, in a report to the Paris Academy of Medicine by Dr. Edgar Berillon, psychologist and authority on mental diseases. He called it '*psychotherapie graphique*,' since the treatment (therapy) combines processes which are both mental (psychic) and physical (graphic). Being intimately interrelated, the two work in unison.

"The efficacy of graphotherapy was tested clinically at the Sorbonne between 1929 and 1931 by two French scientists, Dr. Pierre Janet and Professor Charles Henry." Dr. Janet was professor of psychology at the College de France, and author of *L'Automatisme Psychologique* (Alcan, Paris, 1899-1903). Professor Henry, discoverer of a process to give phosphorescence to zinc sulphide and well-known for his dynamometric experiments, was director of the Sorbonne's Laboratory of Sensations. "In this test," Mr. de Sainte Colombe continues, "I filled the role of consulting psychographologist. Dealing principally with alcoholics and with correcting bad habits in children, the experiment confirmed that the system, intelligently and conscientiously applied, gives positive, impressive results.

"In 1931 a former student of Dr. Janet, Dr. Pierre Menard, who by then had become a distinguished psychology professor, lecturer, and author on medicine and psychology, put the tested technique into practice. In 1948 he brought out his book *La Page d'Ecriture*: *Methode Pratique de Psychotherapie Graphique et Graphologique* (Le Francois, Paris).

"The practice of graphotherapy thus was formally launched in France. In the United States, as far as I can determine, it received no public attention until *Time* Magazine published an article in its April 23, 1956 issue, 'Pen and Pencil Therapy.' The article dealt with the current work of graphotherapist Raymond Trillat with disturbed children in Paris. While it mistakenly suggests that graphotherapy is the discovery of Monsieur Trillat, it nevertheless is informative.

"Trillat uses some devices original with him, but he and all graphotherapists follow, in principle, the same plan. The technique requires the subject to copy a handwriting exercise at least twice a day, morning and night, consciously modifying the script according to instructions supplied by a competent psychographologist.

"To understand graphotherapy, it is necessary to know this psychological principle: a character *flaw* expresses itself exteriorly in bad habits; a character *quality*, in good habits. Laziness, for example, causes the individual consistently to be a late riser, to shirk work, neglect duty. Conscientiousness, on the other hand, is manifested by performance of all tasks expected.... To be indicative of a flaw or a quality, *the behavior must be frequent enough to be termed a habit.*

"Graphotherapy undertakes to break undesirable habits which the hand follows as it writes, replacing them through repetitious exercise with desirable graphic habits. *The hand, if you will, is retrained in specific writing gestures.*

"Handwriting exercises have much in common with the finger exercises employed in learning to play the piano. In the latter case, as long as the pianist must consciously think where to place each finger on the keyboard while reading the music, he proceeds slowly and painfully, making errors. It is only after repetitious practice, when fingers respond automatically and without conscious attention, that the pianist can perform as an accomplished artist. In graphotherapy, the goal is achieved when the desired handwriting change has passed the state of conscious application and imitation, becoming automatic and normal to the hand.

"The time required varies with the individual — it is easier for some people than for others to break a habit. Another factor: How deeply entrenched is the habit, and is it a dominant or minor characteristic? Average cases range from two to six months. The change can be facilitated by faithful application, but it never can be hurried. It takes patience, courage, and the determination to continue as long as necessary to accomplish the aim."

Mr. de Sainte Colombe further said that while in difficult cases it is "indispensable to have the help and supervision of a professional graphotherapist," he knows of no reason "why someone with the intelligence to understand the principles of graphotherapy and to follow instructions should not use it for self-improvement. There is no mystery about it, and anything that can be so enormously helpful should, I believe, have the widest dissemination."

He warns it is important that:

"The elemental personality always be respected. In doing the exercises, retain your natural tempo. If left-handed, continue to write that way, and in your customary script, making only the specific change or changes desired. I sometimes encounter a tendency to revert to carefully made, childlike forms. This is to be avoided....

"Results and cures obtained by this method are absolutely positive. There is growing acceptance among men of science. I am far from being the only dedicated believer in and practitioner of graphotherapy. Though still a relatively small group, a number of highly qualified people practice graphotherapy in various parts of the world. For example, the eminent Robert Olivaus, M.D., uses it in his private practice and at the Bretonneau Hospital in Paris, with remarkable results. And the already-mentioned work of Raymond Trillat among French schoolchildren...."

In his case histories, Mr. de Sainte Colombe included failures and inconclusive results as well as successes because "graphotherapy, like any good remedy, is potent only if the patient stays with it until cured." The French graphotherapist has described his treatment of a college girl who was directed to open the ovals of her writing, elevate the base lines, cross the *t's* firmly, and concentrate on uniform slant. Within a year, he reported, the young woman's writing was transformed, and so was her life — emotional balance had been restored. Psychologist George Melzer, a West Coast behavioral scientist, terms these results "astonishing." John Langdell, M.D., a psychiatrist at San Francisco's Langley Porter Neuropsychiatric Institute, told a reporter he was "a little skeptical about the claims he made for graphotherapy, but I am by no means ready to reject them, either."

Charley Cole, Campbell, California, graphologist, expects "great strides in graphotherapy" in the next decade. "The French have used it for years. Problem children in French schools do writing exercises daily until they fit better into society. It's just a matter of catching up with Europe."

While "Doc" Bunker of the Internatiional Graphoanalysis Society denied the use of intuition in handwriting analysis, Mr. Cole insists "intuition *is* used. But we define intuition as the ability to reach back into the mind and pick out stored knowledge to solve a new and different problem. Just like a computer."

IGS leader V. Peter Ferrara maintains that "evaluation distinguishes scientific graphoanalysis from the occult interpretations of handwriting, all of which are called graphology. It has been said that graphoanalysis is to graphology as astronomy is to astrology." To which Mr. Cole replies, "But graphology is graphology. Graphoanalysis is a coined word."

Prior to 1978, almost all articles appearing in this country on the subject of graphology were in local newspapers or the national "exploitive" press. Such isn't the case today. Almost daily today one can find carefully researched articles on the varied uses of graphology in such outlets as *Journal of Marketing Research*, *American Astrology, Family Circle, Human Behavior, Household, Savvy, Industry Week, German-American Trade News, The A.R.E. Journal*, and even the *Bulletins* of the Bureau of Business Practice, Inc. A very far cry from just a decade ago.

In this book I am attempting to bring a fresh approach to an ancient art, describing in easy-to-grasp language its potential to create peace where there was chaos, health where there was disease, harmony where there was discord.

It doesn't take a protracted series of specialized treatments to learn how to change the attitudes and traits that get us into trouble in day-to-day contact with other members of the human family. The rules are reasonably simple, and they're valid.

How My Life
Was Turned Around

In 1935 I met Robert Lee Clark, lawyer, philosopher, who helped to turn my life around. He helped me to see that the key was to control my emotions—to not react to negative situations. Many changes in my life came about through the counseling of my friend and mentor Professor Clark, which led to achievements and successes I am not bashful about relating:

In 1951 I went to work for Kwikset Lock Company, started by Adolf Schoepe, now head of Fluidmaster, Anaheim. He is a wonderful person, an able executive.

By this time I had built up confidence in myself as a person capable of doing more than secretarial work. Two years later I organized a Toastmistress Club in the Kwikset organization and became its first president. In two years' time I went from the state of stage fright and inability to talk before a group, to winning tri-county "speakoffs" in prepared and impromptu speeches. In 1955 I assisted in the formation of a Soroptimist Club in Anaheim, serving as first vice-president, the next year as president. In 1961 I was one of 11 women in Anaheim to be selected to organize a women's division of the Anaheim Chamber of Commerce, served as first vice-president, and as president the following year. In 1969 I was elected state president of the California Women in Chambers of Commerce.

A BREAK FOR THE DROPOUTS

In Chamber work I was able to persuade the leadership to

seriously look into a vocational program in the school system—a development that has brought recognition to the Orange County educational system and a better life to many young people who were floundering in indecision. Because of my interest in young people, I wanted to head the Chamber's education committee. I had been lecturing to classes on job opportunity and how to prepare for a job; I knew there was a great need for this kind of help. It was agreed this would be my special responsibility, and I went at it with a vengeance in early 1965.

First, we had to study the dropout problem. Why were kids quitting school? Why were they failing in classroom work? Could anything be done about it? On my committee were: the district's top-rated psychologist; the head of the attendance team; the top dog in vocational training (such as it was); a school principal and a teacher from another school in the area; the head of the juvenile section of the Anaheim Police Department; a representative of the Orange County Chamber; a representative of the Orange County School District; and three industrialists. For months we met at breakfast, brainstorming, probing why kids drop out of school. We concluded, for one thing, that these kids just were not college-oriented—they wanted jobs, not more book learning in (for them) dull subjects. And we had to conclude that the educational system was not geared to give such youngsters the training they wanted and needed.

Discouraged and bored, they preferred dropping out to classroom hassle. Among the dropouts were plenty of bright kids who for lack of adult understanding or appreciation of latent abilities and talents, quit rather than fight the system.

So we started studying vocational schools throughout the country. We wrote letters. And I preached vocational education— not a popular concept in the Establishment, I might add. But I *knew* we were on the right track, and persisted. On the board of education was a perceptive, talented individual who caught the vision, and came up with what he termed a 4—4 program to cover mechanics, drafting, carpentry, and plumbing. We sent out signals to industry and, true to the biblical promise *Ask and ye shall receive*, local industries came through nobly. Ford Motor donated a motor for use in the mechanics department; and students spent four hours a day working on it and four hours a day in the classroom. In grammar class the students wrote letters to the Ford people, thanking them for the donation and telling them how it was being used. All their class work was related to that machine. It was the same with the other classes—subjects were correlated with the specific vocational training.

Did the program work? You just know it did! Out of 149 initial dropout students from one Anaheim school, 144 graduated from high school. And the program was arranged so that those who wished could get into a junior college and earn the necessary college credits. But first and foremost, they were equipped to support themselves and engage in useful work that was interesting to them—another way of describing "fulfillment."

Having proved the success of the program, it was only a matter of time until it had been expanded countywide, with a full-time vocation director. This is an example, I say unabashedly, of what one person can do if there is conviction and persistence. People so often ask, "What can I do? I'm only one person." From personal experience I can answer, "You have no idea the power and influence you might exert—if you make up your mind to do it!"

This may be a little off the subject, but not really. It's a close-up of what can happen to a person when the inhibitions, feelings of inadequacy, resentments at society, are replaced by the two words *I can*!

SIX YEARS INTO GRAPHOLOGY

By the time the vocational training adventure had started to develop, I was six years into graphoanalysis. I had had multiple examples that it works; that it can be an instrument not only of balancing one's emotional pattern and creating emotional stasis, but of ferreting out hidden talents and unexpressed inner feelings of the direction a person would like life to take. Not what someone else thinks—never!—but, rather, what lies within *you*, what the Creator has seen fit to endow you with in terms of *serious interest*. That's the first requisite. The other elements for success unfold naturally.

In my own case, one bit of fulfillment led to another during the process of personal growth, and another milestone was reached in 1959 when I started studying handwriting analysis. By this time I had become assistant to the director of industrial relations at

Kwikset, and I wanted to use all the tools available to do the best possible job in hiring and counseling. No one at the office knew about handwriting analysis. I didn't really know what to expect, either. I took the advice of Dr. Milton N. "Doc" Bunker, who told his students, "Don't take my word that handwriting analysis works, prove it." I did just that.

DOC BUNKER PROVED IT TO HIMSELF

This might be the time and place to tell about Doc Bunker's work. He started teaching Gregg shorthand in 1908. As years passed, he was puzzled and disturbed that no matter how diligently he tried to teach and explain and insist on a specific style of letter-formation, students would just as persistently insist on writing in their "natural" style: Some formed large letters, some used extremely small ones, some used wide spacing, others narrow—and he was plain frustrated that he couldn't seem to control it. He happened to be the curious, inquisitive type who had to get answers, so he looked into handwriting analysis. Could this hold the secret? Ultimately he gave up teaching and launched an experiment to determine *for himself* whether handwriting was indeed an index to personality traits. Was it legitimate or bogus? Science or quackery?

Doc Bunker got a sales job and started sending out communications by mail. He tried all sorts of gimmicks to elicit responses, challenging people to react. And as the mail volume grew in response to his queries and probes and prods, the evidence accumulated that handwriting is a guide to personality traits and attitudes just as surely as scent is a guide to a hunting dog. Satisfied that it was not "a lot of hokum," he then developed lessons based on his observations and findings, and launched Graphoanalysis in the 1930s. By 1959, the organization had turned out some 33,000 analysts.

The first or basic course of 18-20 lessons could be completed in a year to 18 months, the graduate or "master" course required up to 2½ years. When I was studying, the cost was about $1,300.

The Bunker approach emphasizes strokes—straight and curves, forward and backward, up and down—and positioning in upper, middle, or lower zones. This concept was not so prevalent in

Europe where graphology had been practiced for centuries and even the American Association of Handwriting Analysts, while recognizing the Bunker concepts, does not rely so heavily on strokes. I find it somewhat more comprehensive, since it also gives attention to margins, distance between lines, distance between words, letter size, and irregularities of letter size — areas in which Europeans have done extensive work.

There is a distinction between *graphology* and *graphoanalysis*: As viewed by a graphoanalyst (a coined word copyrighted by the International Graphoanalysis Society), graphology is a "less accurate forerunner" of graphoanalysis. Graphology is concerned with total formation, or penmanship. Graphoanalysis considers each stroke, or part, that constitutes the total formation.

I PROVED IT TO THE BOSS

My job at Kwikset involved counseling and hiring. We were constantly looking for better people, and it seemed to me I could do a better job for the company and be happier with myself if we screened people with more precision — using a scientific technique, which handwriting analysis is. I was aware that by learning more about the characters of co-workers — those already on the job as well as future employees — I could get pointers in ascertaining likely candidates for upgrading. I knew the people well, and being in the personnel department, had access to their records. This, in fact, is how I proved to myself that handwriting analysis is a valid, reliable means of detecting human traits and attitudes.

No one knew what I was up to; I would not expose myself until I was satisfied as to its merit or worthlessness. As I got into it, I began to see in the employees' handwritings the traits being displayed on the job. They were proving it every day. Exciting? Indeed! But I wasn't so naive as to think I could walk into the boss's office and announce that now we had the answers to all our hiring problems. I didn't have to be a genius to know what sort of response that would bring. So I played it crafty: I started giving talks to groups, getting exposure through newspaper publicity.

I reasoned that if I could persuade the vice-president of sales to let me screen job applicants, using graphology, it would mean money in the bank for the company. So I went to him when I knew what I was talking about, told him, "I have a skill that is important. I believe I can help you. It won't cost you anything — I'm on the job anyway, and I would like to prove it if you'll let me. You can select the handwriting of three of your salesmen. You know I don't have the records, nor any information about their background or performance. Number them, without identifying them, and let me show you." Admitting that he had "nothing to lose," he agreed, and gave me four samples, one at a time. His secretary later told me that No. 4 was his own. Among the habits I had pointed out in his handwriting was that he was "quite a spender, doesn't hang onto money." She just howled when she read it later. 'He's always borrowing money," she said. After No. 4 had been returned to him with my analysis, the vice-president told me, "I'm amazed at what you've done — you have been right to the hair!" And he dictated a letter to my boss that there would be "no hiring without Mrs. Harrison's analysis."

What does this have to do with health? More than one might think at first glance. Industry desperately needs *the right people in the right jobs*. Failure costs the company dollars; it costs the individual oftentimes unknown emotional upset, and eventual physical harm. Unhappiness between people — distorted interpersonal relationships — is a drain on the individuals (though they may not *know* it), as well as on employer resources. Happy people are healthy people. People who can be guided (through analysis of their handwriting) to the career they know they will enjoy, become happy people. Happiness is physical, psychological, emotional health.

Graphology As a Diagnostic Tool

A mass of literature is accumulating as more and more professionals are discovering how an understanding of handwriting can be used in the diagnosis of emotional and physical disorders, and how it can be used in therapy.

One of the articulate and scholarly exponents of this science is Herry O. Teltscher, Ph.D. The following excerpts from his book, *Handwriting — Revelation of Self*, provide insight on observations he has made as to the relative worth of graphology and certain psychological tests to determine personality traits:

"Even though there have been a number of refinements and certain modifications in accordance with results of new investigations, the basic structure of psychographology has remained unaltered. Having utilized handwriting analysis most extensively over the last 25 years, both in research as well as in my daily practice as a psychologist and psychotherapist, my belief in this technique has been strengthened, particularly since the method has so many advantages to offer as compared with other tools of personality evaluation.

"I do not claim handwriting analysis is infallible or that it could not profit from continued validation studies. (Indeed, there have been quite a few.) The same can be said for other methods of personality evaluation, particularly for what psychologists call 'projective techniques,' such as the Rorschach test, or for that matter, psychoanalysis itself. . . .

"The healing profession has shown a growing interest in handwriting analysis — or grapho-diagnosis — in research and in possible practical applications, such as a diagnostic aid. Physicians are becoming more aware of handwriting as a means of detecting ailments not immediately apparent through medical checkups. Research work in the last decade has focused on the early discovery of certain illnesses by the careful study of troubled movements in handwriting. Encouraging studies in the fields of psychosomatic medicine, malignant disease, and neuropsychiatry have been published in recent years. Mental and emotional disturbances have long been diagnosed through handwriting. . . .

"In the hands of the properly educated, trained, and qualified analyst, psychographology can be a most efficient tool, for it operates on the premise that there is no insoluble human relation problem, provided the personality of the other person is correctly understood. It fills a vital need in every field of human contact, and I hope that above all, psychographology will be able to contribute toward solution of the increasingly intricate problems of human adjustment and cooperation in the interest of greater unity, and peace."

IN GOOD SCIENTIFIC STANDING

Although a growing number of practitioners use handwriting analysis as a diagnostic device in mental and physical conditions, the practice still is considered "quackery" in some quarters, as noted by the late Carlton Fredericks, Ph.D., noted nutritionist, author, and lecturer, and visiting professor of nutrition at Fairleigh Dickinson University's School of Education (*Prevention* Magazine May 1973):

"The ABC Network program 'Practice Code' informs writers that their plots must not foster 'superstition or belief' in subjects like graphology. Someone should inform the network that graphology is in good scientific standing as one method of diagnosing certain neurological disorders, and that one of the cancer foundations has invested a great deal of time and money in research in the use of handwriting as a means not only of diagnosing cancer, but of anticipating its onset—as long as 10 years in advance of any of the symptoms currently detectable by medical science. The nervousness of the network with regard to graphology appears to be shared by the orthodoxy in cancer research—accused—by graphologist Alfred Kanfer who developed the handwriting test for cancer—of obstructing his research and blocking publication of papers long ready for press."

USED BY MENTAL CLINIC

The introduction to Nadya Olyanova's *Handwriting Tells*, written by W. Beran Wolfe of the Community Church Mental Hygiene Clinic, New York, reports that handwriting samples are taken of each new patient, and repeated at the time of discharge, for use in comparative scientific research. "The graphological report often discloses psychological or neurological conditions which put the psychiatrist on the track unconsciously hidden by the patient," says Mr. Wolfe. "Nadya Olyanova has demonstrated the keenness of her insight and zeal of her scientific spirit by her clinical research."

BACK PAIN OFTEN PSYCHOSOMATIC

Pain is pain, whether it's "all in the head" or results from a bona fide physical disorder. Back pain often is difficult to pinpoint because the source can defy tests.

Dr. Vert Mooney is doing interesting work with patients at the Problem Back Treatment Center, Rancho Los Amigos Hospital, Downey, California, which he directs.

"Almost anyone with a severe back problem will have a psychological problem," he said. "The pain is very real, but the personality allows it to be magnified."

Also associate clinical professor of orthopedic surgery at the University of Southern California's Medical School in Los Angeles, Dr. Mooney said the goal is to change patients' behavior. Beds are "bugged to determine how much time is spent lying around listlessly. Those who do well are rewarded, those who make no attempt to help themselves are ignored. Rewarding complaints with attention and painkillers just reinforces pain behavior." As of March, 1974, about 80% of approximately 300 patients recovered —through use of "truth drugs," and by keeping close tabs on patients' moods.

Besides the basic tests to determine the cause of back pain, patients receive Pentothal, a "truth drug" that relaxes them enough for doctors to determine how much of the pain is real and how much is subconsciously imagined.

"Some patients then are given painkilling medication," Dr. Mooney said. "But unknown to the patient, the painkilling ingredients are slowly phased out. The patient believes the medicine is still reducing the pain."

Graphotherapy—a French Discovery

The link between emotional imbalance and physical disease has been documented by so many, so often, that it is "no longer debatable."

Among the books that have created public awareness of this are *Release from Nervous Tension* by David Harold Fink, M.D.; *How to Live 365 Days a Year* by John Schindler, M.D., and *It's a Grand Life*, written and published in 1969 by Frank B. Hamilton, Ph.D.

H.K. Flanders Dunbar, M.D., of Presbyterian Hospital, New York, demonstrated clinically many times that unpleasant emotions produce changes in body tissue.

"In some cases, stomach ulcer is a result of interbrain disturbance," writes Dr. Fink. "Heart disease may be another." Dr. Fink reports the case of a woman with such a severe case of mucous colitis that blood in the stool was sometimes observed. Under his sympathetic questioning, he learned she had a "stern, cold husband," and that three years earlier she had yielded to an indiscretion with another man and feared her husband might learn about it. "She wanted to tell her husband but was afraid. She blamed him for driving her to the act, yet would have liked to have hurt him by letting him know, since she was suffering for lack of love. At any rate, eventually there was a scene, a reconciliation, and the mucous colitis of three years' duration ceased at once."

Virtually every known human trait—fear, uncertainty, elation, inconsistency, deviousness, resentment, jealousy, insecurity, apprehension—the list is long—is reflected in the handwriting of the afflicted person. All these attitudes result in stress transmitted via the nervous system to vital organs. Dr. Hamilton places heavy emphasis on emotionally induced stress in his book *It's a Grand Life*.

The stress-disease relationship, of course, has been documented clinically for many years by Hans Selye, M.D., of Montreal.

Many emotionally induced illnesses respond not to outside or external modalities (surgery, irradiation, drugs), but rather to resources of the affected individual: Your own will, mind, spiritual outlook. Help is available, indeed, but the healing must start with you.

GRAPHOTHERAPY IN FRANCE

Now what has all this to do with handwriting, you ask? As noted by Paul de Sainte Colombe in the introductory chapter, the practice of graphotherapy was formally launched in France nearly half a century ago. Dr. Edgar Berillon did the early research with his *psychotherapie graphique* technique, and Dr. Pierre Janet and Professor Charles Henry clinically tested it between 1929 and 1931. Then came the contribution of Dr. Pierre Menard, student of Dr. Janet, whose work was published in book form in 1948.

TO KNOW ONESELF

In his *Grapho-Therapeutics*, Dr. Colombe says:

"How is graphology useful? In what areas may it be applied? First and foremost, graphology answers the need to know oneself. It has been said that a man has three characters: The one he exhibits, the one he actually has, and the one he *thinks* he has.

"Few can accurately discover all the truth about themselves without help, since it is obscured by a number of things, not the least of which is the strong tendency to deceive ourselves. And while it may sometimes be easier and more comfortable to hide from the truth than face it, it is neither wise nor profitable, and often is downright disastrous.

"Like the body, the personality can become sick, and it never helps to just let it go. Then there are the unfortunate souls who suffer all their lives from terrible fears, entirely unfounded, and the many who, unaware of their natural aptitudes and lacking professional orientation, are square pegs trying desperately and hopelessly to fit themselves into round holes. It is bad enough to be misunderstood, but to not understand oneself is intolerable, and foolishly unnecessary."

...AND OTHERS

"It is self-evident that to acquaint ourselves with the real, underlying character of those with whom we associate intimately or in any other way, is to provide ourselves with a valuable safeguard against heartache and losses. Marriage need no longer be a gamble when two people can discover beforehand what each is truly like. Family relationships usually are improved, and friction reduced, when understanding replaces emotional thinking and attitudes. Graphology can enable us to encourage worthwhile friends and avoid false ones. Parents can guide children more wisely if aware of their innate tendencies—and they ought to know all there is to know about a nurse or babysitter before trusting their offspring to that person.

"Employers can avoid hiring dishonest, incompetent or badly adjusted employees. Conversely, they can avoid firing a potentially good employee who may be showing up poorly due to some temporary disruption in personal life...."

DIAGNOSTIC TOOL

"In psychiatry, all types of abnormality—from slight mental and emotional disturbances to schizophrenia, paranoia, and sexual deviations—are discernible in handwriting. This makes graphology a remarkable diagnostic tool, permitting the practitioner to go directly to the root of the trouble. It enables him to chart personality changes under treatment, and thus determine if correct results are being obtained. And by shortening the time of diagnosis and perhaps treatment, the patient is spared not only expense but he may avoid one of the harmful side effects of psychiatric treatment: Prolonged self-examination and analysis of the most minute thought and act tends to turn a person inward until all other interests disappear....

"Graphology now is taught in several colleges and universities (in France) as part of the psychiatry course, yet many practicing psychiatrists know nothing about it and reject its use. These doctors rely on the Rorschach (ink-blot) test which cannot begin to give what handwriting does—and certainly not with nearly the degree of accuracy. With Rorschach, too many different interpretations are posssible to make it reliable, and the patient may know sufficient psychology to mislead the tester.

"Handwriting is full of health clues which clearly reveal disorders of heart, stomach, joints, and the nervous and glandular systems. It also reveals epilepsy.

"Geriatricians find graphopathology enormously helpful in treatment of the aged because it permits them to distinguish between ordinary senility and mental unbalance, between the normal physical weakening which comes with old age, and actual disease."

DETECTING CANCER: KANFER

"The newest development in the area of pathology has been detecting cancer from handwriting, which the late Alfred Kanfer did after 30 years of research, pursued first in his native Vienna, then, after becoming a refugee from Hitler, at the Strang Clinic for Preventive Medicine in New York where from 1963 until his death in 1974 he received aid and encouragement from the Handwriting Institute. Since the medical profession is notoriously slow to embrace radical innovations—and they are right to be cautious—doctors scoffed in the beginning, although they could not quite figure out how Mr. Kanfer, by examining fountain-penned handwriting under a 50-power projection microscope, could achieve a score for accuracy of between 70% and 80%. The odds against doing this by pure chance are about one in ten million. He measured variations in the thickness of strokes.

"For a long time, Mr. Kanfer himself could not explain why cancer should manifest in handwriting or why it should show up there months and even years before it could be detected medically. Then medical research turned up data which suggests there is a neuromuscular deterioration detectable in malignancy patients, and this, of course, would affect handwriting . . . ."

PERSONALITY FLAWS

After discussing the use of graphology in criminal investigations, Dr. Colombe observes:

"The treatment of personality and character flaws through deliberately made changes in the handwriting offers a whole new field for the graphologist. The possibilities for giving quick, effective help where needed are almost boundless in dealing with the myriad problems growing out of character defects. In the case of children, where character is in the process of being formed, graphotherapy is particularly effective—one can even say ideal. And this is true whether the child is 'disturbed,' delinquent, or just an average youngster needing guidance to arrest undesirable tendencies and to develop desirable, sturdy characteristics to see him through life and permit him to make the most of his potentials."

SKIN DISORDERS: DR. LOO

What the French physicians started has been continued by others—not a stampede of doctors to utilize the technique, of course—but, nonetheless, doctors with inquisitive, open minds have applied the principles and the technique itself. And remarkable results are being reported.

Acknowledging that he was quite aware "there would be scoffers and ridiculers," Dr. Cyrus W. Loo, a medical doctor in Hawaii, has used graphotherapy to clear up skin disorders. This dermatologist said that in addition to the medicine chest, he has found handwriting analysis "extremely valuable" in his practice, particularly in determining the emotional state of patients afflicted with one of the several skin diseases falling within the category of neurodermatitis. Emotions, he says, cause more than 50% of skin ailments in patients he has treated. "Handwriting is brainwriting," he asserts. "It can't be disguised, and it reveals much of a person's character and personality." It also discloses irritability, extreme sensitivity, domineering tendencies, anxiety, impatience, impulsiveness, resentment—all of which are in the self-destruct category.

He explains the medical application of graphotherapy thusly:

"Many skin disorders are caused or aggravated by emotional components. An understanding of the patient's personality is of extreme importance in order to effect proper treatment. Dermatologists need rapid and valid means of assessing personality. When the degree of severity of the emotional disturbance is known, a decision can be made whether to refer to a psychiatrist or treat the patient oneself, utilizing a more simple psychological approach."

Dr. Loo obtains handwriting samples from those with severe neurodermatitis—skin disorders traceable to nerves. After analyzing the specimen to uncover personality traits, he categorizes the patient into treatment routines.

"By means of handwriting analysis," he continues, "one can detect with accuracy hidden traits of character which may not even be known to the outside world. There is a correlation between writing and personality, and when a personality change occurs, the writing reflects it." He tells about the patient whose skin eruptions he traced through her handwriting to "aggressive tendencies." During counseling he learned there was subconscious enmity toward the mother. He was trying to correct a skin condition "while she was eating her heart out!" When the repressed animosity was identified, and graphotherapy instituted, the causative factor was eliminated by means of handwriting exercises, and the skin cleared. This doctor views handwriting as "a useful tool also for screening applicants for a job, in choosing marital partners, vocational counseling, police work, understanding 'problem children,' credit counseling, adoption placement, and detecting disturbed mental conditions."

PRODUCTS OF FEAR

Among the fear traits that may be uncovered are *jealousy* (fear of not being loved); *sensitivity to criticism* (fear of disapproval); *self-underestimation* (fear of failure); *self-consciousness* (fear of ridicule); *indecisiveness* (fear of finality); *stinginess* (fear of want); *ultraconservatism* (fear of change); *timidity* (fear of social activities).

Nervous irritability can lead to asthma, allergies, and ulcers.

Fear causes excessive amounts of sugar to be secreted into the blood — nature's survival mechanism to provide quick added strength and endurance. Continual stimulation, however, results in low blood sugar, resulting in hyperfunction of the islets of Langerhans which, in turn, lowers the blood sugar to create hypoglycemia, a common disease in modern society.

Fear, a mental process, pictures vividly a dreaded disease or situation, and unless neutralized these images materialize — self-fulfilling prophecy, the psychologists call it.

Constant criticism of others is another disease-producer: Negative, inharmonious thoughts actually generate unnatural deposits in the blood that settle in the joints, causing what we know as rheumatism or arthritis.

Unwanted growths may originate in such emotions as *fear, jealousy, hatred, inability to forgive*. This last-named trait is one of the most prolific causes of disease. It hardens the arteries, and also affects eyesight. *Anger* blurs vision, sets in motion a chain of reactions culminating in injection of toxins into the bloodstream. Most problems, mental and physical, originate with fears in the subconscious. Graphotherapy has a significant potential for helping those so afflicted.

KEY TO HAPPINESS: BLOODWORTH

In her *Key to Yourself*, Dr. Venice Bloodworth comments:

"The primary cause of every disease is mental or spiritual discord, and the only permanent basis for health and happiness is mental and spiritual harmony.

"Every emotion and mental attitude creates after its kind. Intense anger with destructive intentions attracts physical injury to yourself, while fear, hate, anger, unkind criticism produce rheumatism, lumbago, headache, stomach trouble, to name a few. You may gain a certain measure of relief through medication, but permanent relief is not possible until mental discord is removed. . . for pain is an inharmonious mental vibration registering distress in the cells. Anger causes high blood pressure with its kindred ills. Harsh, angry, destructive thoughts bring accidents, burns, broken bones. Violence is caused by violent emotions, and the fear of violence.

"Every phase of hate, anger, prejudice, criticism, jealousy, envy, greed, is the expression of fear in some form. Jealousy is fear of losing a loved one, or position in the social or economic structure, and is caused by a lack of self-confidence to hold your own.

"Envy is an expression of weakness.... The person possessing what we see as desirable character, envies no one.

"Greed is a highly developed sense of want. Many who pile up great fortunes did not possess the comforts of childhood.

"Jealousy, envy, greed, grief, are the precursors to liver and kidney trouble, constipation, biliousness. Grief, hate, and opposition bring on symptoms of heart disease, arteriosclerosis, general congestion. Heart trouble is a specific result of mental opposition....

"Children are the most helpless sufferers from adverse thoughts since the young sensitive mind receives impressions without protection...."

Dr. Bloodworth uses this quotation from Psalms to open her chapter on "Disease": *Bless Jehovah, O my soul, who forgiveth all thine iniquities, who healeth all thy diseases.*

1,000 FIRMS USING GRAPHOANALYSIS

The Wall Street Journal reporter David M. Elsner wrote in June 1974 that "although most scientists doubt the validity of handwriting analysis, an estimated 1,000 United States firms employ consulting analysts, double the number five years ago, analysts say."

The story quotes Robert W. Buckenberg who is vice-president of sales, Guaranty Reserve Life Insurance, Hammond, Indiana, and who employs graphologist Nicholas R. Burczyk, Lansing, Michigan, to analyze the handwriting of employees and potential employees: "I'd say the handwriting test is accurate 80% of the time. Mr. Burczyk told us that one of our men was in poor health. The man then told us he was having a respiratory problem that he hadn't mentioned to anyone. He went to a doctor who found he had diabetes."

Another doctor, said *The Wall Street Journal* story, "who believes 'there's definitely some substance to it,' is Dr. John Lee, professor of clinical psychiatry at Chicago Medical School, who has been studying the relationship between handwriting and personality for more than a year. Dr. Lee says he has begun comparing handwriting analyses of psychiatric patients with observations made by their doctors. 'There are correlations, but it's too early to say anything definite yet.'"

SIGNIFICANT WORK IN SPAIN

But Dr. Joaquin Alegret, a senior lecturer on the faculty of medicine at the University of Madrid, who teaches "The Psychology of Handwriting" at the university, is further along in his thinking—and his conclusions. In a story dated January 21, 1973, he told *The National Enquirer* that 95% of the patients treated by the science have been cured of psychological illnesses— and it can work just as well in some cases of organic disease.

"In some cases," he said, "the new science of graphology can be more useful than psychiatry. Its main benefit is speed. You may need hundreds of hours of psychoanalysis before you uncover the unconscious mind. But I have found that two days' study of a page of handwriting can lead straight to certain hidden tendencies. The main advantage is that the patient does not know what you are seeing from the handwriting. In psychoanalysis, an intelligent patient can see what the analyst is getting at and create barriers. Graphology is far more useful in diagnosing cases of extreme depression, kleptomania, and suicidal tendencies than psychiatry."

Dr. Alegret continued, "While this part of the potential benefits of graphology is still in its infancy, I do have case histories of purely organic cures of such ailments as throat disease, acute stomach trouble—and above all, nervous diseases. Several months ago, for example, I treated a patient who complained of continual headaches. I made the routine tests for sinus, but there was no problem there. Then I asked him to write two paragraphs. After studying the handwriting in detail, I could tell him he had a pathological tendency for suicide through fear of failure in his office. He scoffed. But I asked him to try to give his handwriting more definition—to cross the *t* correctly, and to clarify the capital letters. *After three weeks, the man's handwriting became better, his headaches lessened, and so did his tendency toward suicide. He is now awaiting a promotion.*"

The doctor explained that "by instructing a patient on how he should change the handwriting, we can give him new psychological reflexes. The patient works on altering what has been natural throughout life, and in so doing, corrects character defects which have brought illness."

The Enquirer story ended by quoting a colleague at the University of Madrid: "Dr. Alegret's studies have vast importance in the sociological field—mainly because ordinary people can have the benefit of some sort of psychiatry without paying the enormous sums necessary for sessions on a couch. I believe completely in what he is doing. This is not only a breakthrough in medicine, but in sociology as well."

INJURY AFFECTS HANDWRITING

Analyst Antonia Klekoda, in a story on February 24, 1974, in *The National Tattler*, described how injury or recent surgery affects handwriting:

"It modifies it or radically changes it," she says. "For example, actor John Wayne's crippled autograph contains his awareness of his missing lung, due to cancer surgery. (This is seen by noting the indentation of the *h* as it relates to and 'marks' the missing lung. A similar indentation in the writing of lung-damaged patients was discovered by psychologists in a tuberculosis sanitarium at the turn of the century.)

"Another indication of poor physical health is ragged writing. Unlike the indentations, which note damage already done, ragged specimens of writing can be useful to physicians as an aid to preventive medicine. Actor Johnny 'Tarzan' Weissmuller's script is an excellent example. The actor, who reportedly suffers from heart problems, has an *l* indentation.

"When Admiral Horatio Nelson lost his right arm, he learned to write with his left hand quite legibly. However, he carried a 'picture' of the dismemberment on the right side of his *t*'s which marked the crippled part of his body."

Priests and Nuns Use It

There was a time when handwriting analysis was considered a gift from the Powers of Darkness—with origins in the occult—and thus was shunned by those professing belief in Judeo-Christian teachings. But no more. Its emergence as a useful tool in discerning personality traits, when used by trained individuals with integrity, has erased that image. And if there are any still who would challenge this thesis—do they know about the growing use of graphology in the Catholic Church? Rather an exciting story—really!

In 1964 Macmillan published a book, *The Saints Through Their Handwriting*, by a well-known Italian graphologist, Father Girolamo M. Moretti, O.F.M. It started as a study, encouraged by Father Fernando Vesprini who now says, "It will not be possible in the future to write the biography of a saint without a handwriting analysis. It prepares the background on which the halo rests."

Father Moretti analyzed the handwritings of 32 unidentified (to him) saints. Upon completion of the analyses, his findings were compared with the characters of the saints as shown in definitive biographies. Father Moretti's conclusions on emotions, intelligence, and personalities, it turned out, were virtually identical with appraisals by biographers.

There are a number of priests and sisters in the United States, and some in Canada, whose work in the field of graphology has been accorded publicity.

In Canada, the Rev. J. Wilfrid Cyr of Trois Rivieres, Quebec, has become known for his activity in promoting handwriting analysis as a useful adjunct to psychological testing.

In the United States, Mother M. Cecilia Koehler, O.S.U., past mother superior of the order, in 1961 earned the first "Graphologist of the Year" award from fellow members of the International Graphoanalysis Society. She lectures on the handwriting of the predelinquent, and how to develop desirable personality traits in teenagers. She has done writing analysis studies for members of the clergy from as far away as Guatemala, and has worked with the Papal Volunteers for Latin America, analyzing the handwritings of candidates for PAVLA. She looks for such traits as emotional balance, ability, interest areas, character stamina, will to achieve, affability, ability to work with others and social qualities.

"A skilled handwriting analyst looks for and evaluates 110 to 120 different elements," she told Patricia Coleman, author of a story in *Extension*. "One trait by itself is absolutely meaningless."

Others in the growing band of Catholic clergy trained in handwriting analysis who are in the forefront of practitioners intent on removing handwriting analysis from "a cloud of mystery" and in building for it a professional image, are the Reverend Anthony J. Becker of St. Charles, Illinois, 1976 president of the American Association of Handwriting Analysts and one of its ardent spokespersons; the Reverend Norman J. Werling, O. Carm., of Oakland, New Jersey, who like Father Becker is a qualified psychologist and specialist in educational testing and interpretation; Sister Bernice, Ad. P.P.S., East St. Louis, Illinois; Sister Mary Theophane of Albuquerque, New Mexico; Mother Patricia, O.C.D., Carmelite Monastery, Boston; and Sister Augustine, St. James School, Augusta, Kansas.

In Paola, Kansas, the sisters at Ursuline Academy are trained observers of handwriting, using the knowledge of what handwriting says about a person to gain better understanding of their students. Each sister has taken at least one basic course in handwriting analysis; many have qualified for certification after advanced training. And even before becoming a sister, these nuns are introduced to handwriting study—their handwriting was analyzed when they were candidates for the Order, once before receiving the habit, and again before making final vows. That's routine procedure.

'We use handwriting as a guide, one more tool in screening and getting to know applicants," says Mother Cecilia. "Later it helps guide us in placing sisters in positions to which they are most fitted."

Mother Cecilia frequently conducts classes in handwriting analysis for local townspeople. "Teachers aren't the only ones who benefit from an understanding of handwriting; parents also profit. They face tremendous pressures and problems raising children. Knowledge of handwriting analysis can be of value in performing that job."

Father Becker, with a Ph.D. in educational psychology, is counselor, chaplain and faculty member at St. Dominic College in St. Charles. One of his most valuable counseling tools is handwriting analysis. "Like a movie camera or tape recorder," he says, "handwriting is captured behavior. A fingerprint tells *who* a person is. Handwriting tells *what* he is, when you know how to interpret the signs."

Father Becker is among the leaders in the writing analysis movement working to open up approved and controlled study in the field, which he readily admits has been "too much restricted." A partial reason for slow progress in winning wider acceptance of handwriting analysis is the "cold war" between two groups differing on the most effective technique. Wrote Ms. Coleman:

"Is it the way of graphology? Or is it the methods of graphoanalysis? Father Becker thinks the answer need not be one or the other, but tolerance of both approaches, and more research and pooling of information. (Graphologists recognize certain character traits through formation and combination of letters, whereas graphoanalysts reveal the individual by analyzing strokes.)

"Says Father Becker: 'I consider handwriting analysis an added diagnostic tool to psychology. By no means does it replace other recognized treatment or techniques. It has a function all its own—to help x-ray a problem. What writing does actually is to crack open the subconscious. Like intelligence tests, its analysis is one other effort to help assess the human personality. It should be taken seriously, too, by the professional community, as handwriting analysis on the whole proves 80% to 85% accurate—a sit-up-and-take-notice score for any testing method.'"

Father Becker likes to speak on the subject, and talks about it with seminarians, hospital administrators, and members of civic, educational, and social organizations. While a skilled analyst can make a brief personality profile from a signature and a line or two of writng, several pages of samples at different times usually are required for a comprehensive scientific evaluation, he says, since one's writing varies according to mood and circumstances. "Results are best when the subject does not know he is writing for analysis," he adds.

THIS PRIEST HELPS YOUNG ADDICTS

For Father Werling, a master graphoanalyst at St. Cecilia's Rectory, Englewood, New Jersey, handwriting analysis is the first step in his counseling—whether it's determining a married couple's compatibility, or learning if there's still hope for a young person hooked on drugs.

Interviewed by Sherrie Moran of the *Fort Lauderdale News* during a convention of Florida Graphoanalysts, Inc., Father Werling said that by studying the handwriting of young addicts "we can see how far they've gone. If there's a lot of hope, the judge can sentence them but require them to get medical help. If the judge assigns this, the state pays for it. So it's my gruesome task to have eight or ten kids a week sentenced."

Father Werling cited these "common traits" in the handwriting of young people involved in drugs:

"They're usually the athletic type, and intelligent—frustrated kids who don't know what to do with their brains, and energy. [His voice rose in frustrated anger as he recalled seeing the tragedy repeated in so many lives.] Others, who don't have the energy and are fairly dull, just kind of sit. Those who want to be doing something don't have an outlet. From their writing we can tell their vocational possibilities."

As a counselor Father Werling does "a lot of private vocational counseling" with students, and "handwriting helps me do the job better. The time for individual conferences during retreats is so short, and students generally are hesitant to open up quickly. I'm interested in getting at causes, and handwriting helps me get there fast.

"When a person's handwriting changes suddenly, it's a sign something is wrong. I would like to see teachers trained to detect these signs. Often, the change in writing is the first indication of a serious emotional problem, or even the start of a drug experience.

Teachers also could spot emotionally disturbed children at the beginning of the year, almost as quickly as thumbing through a stack of papers they've written. The papers could be taken to the counselor with the request, 'Here, do something for these kids now, not at the end of the year.'"

Father Werling and a New Jersey Serra chapter collaborated on a research project to establish status for handwriting analysis in screening candidates for the priesthood and religious life. As part of the documented case study, he analyzed 2,000 samples of nuns' handwritings to chart an "ideal personality," to set down some temperamental trait aptitudes for evaluation. He says writing analysis actually proves more accurate in furnishing much-needed guidelines than standard aptitude or psychological testing methods now available.

This priest even turns the technique on himself. "About a year ago I noticed my writing had become very shaky, very small (a sign of tension). I noticed it one day so I went back over my writing for a couple of weeks. Then I told my boss goodbye and went off for a couple of weeks. I just hadn't realized how much things had been piling up."

While a limited sample of writing can indicate a serious emotional problem, Father Werling said a bona fide analysis is not done without several samples. "With only one sample, all we have is what the person was like at the time he wrote it. With several samples, ingrained characteristics can be detected. Handwriting is expressive behavior. We don't analyze the ink on the paper, we recreate the motion the person went through to make this writing. The ink line has frozen this emotion."

To illustrate, he pulled out a piece of paper on which a friend had written his signature six times, three with eyes open, three with them closed. A series of circles and lines comparing the signatures showed uniformity of spacing and motion in all six signatures. "It also illustrated how exacting a science graphoanalysis really is," commented Sherrie Moran.

"It's impossible to estimate how many elements there are in a page of writing," continued Father Werling. "Let's say there are five million. These include angles, dots, slants, curve lines, straight lines."

The fact that two books on the best-seller list were about analyzing doodles, and authored by doctors, indicated to him that handwriting analysis finally will be taken seriously as a psychological tool. "From doodling it's one easy step to handwriting. I don't try to oversell it, it's not the whole answer of course, but it's one more technique.

"The way a person walks, talks, and gestures all reveal points about personality, just as handwriting does. But only recently have American psychologists begun to become interested in it. Before, everything was the white rat, stimulus-response. Now we know there's more to psychosomatic medicine than glands and muscles. The personality is what we have to study. Until we come up with more knowledge about personality, we're at a dead end."

Ms. Moran continued: "When Father Werling's getting into his favorite topic, it's an easy transition from the serious side to the intriguing thought of learning about the character of famous persons. He told of a reporter who gave him samples of three persons' writings, without revealing identities.

"'The first I thought was very artistic, with great organization, well-balanced, a fine personality, disciplined, but rather snobbish. It turned out to be Bess Myerson.

"The second person I thought was very timid and idealistic. It was Martin Luther King, Jr. It was a letter he had written the reporter who had covered him for a month. The reporter told me that when Mr. King was alone he was almost like a timid rabbit. The third sample was the reporter's."

"Father Werling has done a developmental study of John Kennedy's writing from childhood through the presidency. 'Until he found himself, he was lots of problems to himself and others. It was in law school that he found himself and knew what he wanted.'

"Queen Victoria was in the habit of dotting *i*'s with a circle. Jackie Onassis' writing has this trait. I tell people circles over *i*'s indicate a woman who wants to own an island.'

"Another time he was given a sample of writing and told it was that of a 15-year-old boy. 'It had great maturity, drive, organization, leadership. I said if that's really a 15-year-old boy, I want to know what happens to him. Then they told me it was Franklin Roosevelt's writing at 15.

"When I look at mine, I could cry. The base line is all over the place, which means my moods are all over the place. And that's me,' he laughed.

"Then he showed how, when he writes the *g* at the end of his name he brings the tail down in a straight line, with no loop. 'That's a hermit—that's me.'"

$$q \quad g \quad g \quad g \quad g \quad g \quad g$$
$$1 \quad 2 \quad 3 \quad 4 \quad 5 \quad 6 \quad 7$$

"Loops at the end of letters indicate sociability—from the hermit (no. 1) to 'someone who likes to be in a football stadium with 30,000 people' (no. 7). Father Werling, a No. 1, joked, 'I wonder if the Pope changed the rule about priests marrying, if I'd become a No. 7?'"

Secrets In Your
Child's Handwriting

As a windmill responds to air currents, our nervous and emotional systems respond to external environment. Thus, when mother and dad are in perpetual conflict, it rubs off on the children. They don't miss much, even as babies. And when love expressed at the altar has eroded—when criticism and harangue has replaced harmony in the parent relationship—the waves create emotional upset leading to behavioral *and physical* disturbances in Kate and Johnny. There's just too much documentation of this to allow for argument. It's an irrefutable psychological fact. And not the easiest thing to acknowledge if we're parents, right?

The youngster who through no fault of her own inherits a brutalized homelife cannot be herself. She is not free. This child represses emotions, holds back joy or tears, knowing it might provoke a parental outburst. Abused, beaten, and denied, she is likely to wind up on the street, in jail, or in a mental hospital. This personality is described as "neurotic, psychotic."

Standing out like red flags to the graphologist are certain predictable characteristics in the handwriting of this unfortunate child. The trained analyst spots severe repression, absence of movement, along with these familiar signals: Variable slant; uneven (moody) base lines; tightly closed ovals in middle zone; awkward, twisted letter formations; unfinished strokes—all of which add up to an unhealthy child!

Happiness is more comp than comfort, enjoyment, satisfaction. It is more sere

GRAPHOTHERAPEUTICS TO THE RESCUE!

The treatment of personality and character flaws through deliberately made changes in handwriting produces quick, effective help—particularly among children.

Paul de St. Colombe describes the work of Raymond Trillat in France, and his extraordinary success correcting children's problems through the use of exercises to correct handwriting flaws. Here are a few suggestions resulting from Mr. Trillat's experiences:

Introverts have difficulty connecting letters. The *timid* squeeze letters together. Since he had proved to himself that mental disturbances and emotional problems show plainly in handwriting, he developed writing exercises designed to give children a sense of *continuity*, *creation*, and *equilibrium*. In overcoming negative characteristics, he said a child first must develop a feeling for *rhythm*, *melody*, and *harmony*.

He discovered that neurotic children, some of them stutterers, do not follow through. Some could not open a door with a single gesture, instead pulling it in a series of hesitant, jerky movements. He starts such children out with a series of connected e e e e e 's.

eeeee   eeeee   eeeee

Then he teaches them to move on to variations:

elle ppo elle ppo

For the exceptionally nervous child, he designed special "sedative" exercises: e flow e flow etc.

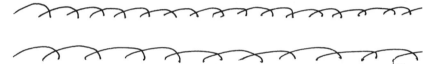

For the unstable, a series of plaits to develop "continuity in a discontinued movement."

Those who squeeze letters practice broad sweeping motions:

And those who spread letters too much through lack of a sense of harmony are trained to develop a consciousness of space and balance by writing:

Later each child is encouraged to find his own creative personality by forming the letters individually.

Equilibrium is developed by slanting the writing in one direction, making letters uniform in size.

In a ten-year period Mr. Trillat treated more than 600 children, and reports helping or curing 5 out of 6. He found that emotional problems lead to illegibility, and illegibility leads to more emotional problems — a vicious circle.

Milton N. Bunker, founder of the International Graphoanalysis Society, developed a number of important exercises in corrective handwriting. His contribution to graphotherapy includes these exercises:

Cramped and compressed writing, combined with heavy pressure, invariably is related to anxieties and worries, so he taught students to open up, spread their writing, thus:

Children whose *t*-bars were "weak," an indicator of lack of will and planning ability, practiced making heavy *t*-bars:

t   t   t   t   t   t   t   t   t

To develop self-reliance, they were taught to inscribe heavy lines below the signature, ending the final stroke rightward:

John Smith

For mental growth:

To develop imagination:

llll   hhhh   kkkk
gggg   y   y   y   gggg

To overcome timidity and conservatism:

WHAT ONE TEACHER HAS DONE

Among my students was an elementary school teacher who, through handwriting therapy and counseling, has accomplished astonishing character changes with "problem children" who have not suffered brain damage.

She is grapholgist Betty Lee Kesten, who teaches in the Downey, California, school system. Other teachers have reported success with graphotherapy, but Mrs. Kesten's record is outstanding. Here are some of the traits these youngsters overcame through patient use of corrective handwriting:

List: Limited attention span. Inability to concentrate. Handwriting "loaded" with errors, Inability to maintain logical flow of thought—characterized by small letters of varying size. Slow to comprehend ideas. Self-consciousness. Self-underestimation. Jealousy. Overaggressiveness, Irritability, Temper tantrums. Repression. Timidity.

The teachers' goal, achieved in a high percentage of cases, is to engender greater enthusiasm, instill a feeling of self-reliance, a desire to develop imagination, and eagerness to learn.

Working daily with children, positive results were achieved by gradually eliminating negative traits from the handwriting. Through numerous exercises, including more uniform spacing and better organization, youngsters are freed of tension and frustrations. Examples of corrective exercises:

For concentration and memory improvement:

To stimulate self-confidence and ambition (strong *t*-bars):

For openness in writing, circular motion:

For rhythm and graceful movement, wavy strokes:

To promote fluency of thought, interesting combinations of *f* and *g*:

Teachers using graphology to pinpoint a child's emotional problems, then instituting graphotherapy, have been gratified with results.

Mrs. Kesten says children usually begin cursive writing (letters joined) when they reach third grade, and that about four months are required to master it *if they are free of fears and hangups.* However, she says, if a child is not yet writing, it still is possible to analyze pictures drawn by the youngster, since the "inner self" is being projected on paper. Language disability and disorganized handwriting go hand-in-hand, she has discovered, since writing is more difficult to master than verbal communication. In writing, the child must form a mental image of each letter, than transfer it to paper. In the process, he actualizes his total environment and the external forces affecting him.

"Several basic factors must be considered," says Mrs. Kesten, "when analyzing a child's handwriting: 1) Firmness, and evenness of stroke. 2) Depth (pressure), indicates attunement with color sense, and a sense of 'feeling' or 'belonging' in one's environment. 3) Correct, clear writing, without blotches, letters open where they should be open, closed when they should be closed, are all important.

"4) Organization of one's writing and mental development have much in common. 5) Round structures indicate pliable character, but when overdone, we see the older child as too pliant. This trait should not extend beyond adolescence. 6) The rigid child (opposite of pliable-roundness in writing) is difficult for a teacher to work with. 7) It is important to recognize optimism in writing, and 8) angularity—a window to the individual's reasoning ability. This alone tells the skilled graphologist more about the child than anything else, because there are children with neurological impairment—basically bright—who do their academic work but aren't able to *use* the knowledge. Many of these children find it impossible to learn language, spelling, and the written word, but are mechanical geniuses, skilled with their hands. I have worked with children in the Educationally (and emotionally) Handicapped (E.H.) program who apparently learn, but when required to use the knowledge, simply cannot do it. The input comes out highly disorganized. And significantly, many are very kind, thoughtful, and try diligently to do the classwork.

"There is urgent need for changes in dealing with the

handicapped child who cannot learn but is able to work with the hands—often a mechanical whiz. The youngsters, experiencing one defeat after another, but nevertheless, advanced from grade to grade in a system which seems to ignore their needs, too often end up as pathetic misfits, and not infrequently, as suicides, unable to cope in a society in which no one seems to understand how to help them beyond a certain point."

SISTER AUGUSTINE USES IT

An avowed advocate of handwriting analysis in the classroom is Sister M. Augustine Weilert, Order of Adorers of the Blood of Christ, and principal in St. James School, Augusta, Kansas.

President of the Kansas Chapter of International Graphoanalysis Society and winner of the 1968 Coop award for attracting the most new students to the professional study of handwriting analysis, Sister Augustine told the *Wichita Eagle and Beacon* (October 1969) that she "wouldn't take a million dollars for my knowledge of handwriting. It's a privilege as well as a responsibility to possess the master key to a child's personality, or let's say—a child's world."

Besides her position as principal, Sister Augustine is a certified school psychologist and fulltime teacher of third through fifth grades. She reminds us that graphoanalysis is not a fortune-telling device, but an accepted scientific system of identifying the character and personality of an individual through study of the handwriting.

"When we look at the writing of a young boy or girl we see in the strokes the influence the home has exerted on the personality of the writer. Many children suffer from basic needs and rights, become frustrated, rebellious or withdrawn, depending on their nature.

"We don't analyze from the content of the writing. I rarely read the words. It is in the strokes and shape, the heaviness or lightness of letters. For instance—unwholesome fear can be seen in the heavy compressed *m*, *n*, and *h*. Some strokes show deep hurts, withdrawal, frustration. We might see deprivation in the retraced strokes, or timidity in indefinite or yielding strokes.

"But more important are the resulting characteristics in these deprived little ones—such as persistent stealing, not for material gain but to satisfy emotional needs...aggressiveness, deceit, jealousy, fear of not being loved, clannishness, vanity, air castles, and learning inhibitions. All these, if known by teacher or counselor, can be a tremendous help as a guiding tool.

"If all teachers were graphoanalysts—and we hope some day they will be—much good could be done to alleviate children's problems by working with the parents.

"Handwriting has been called brainwriting, and it is. Whether you write with a pen between your teeth, the crook of your arm, or between your toes, the strokes instantly reveal frame of mind. If a child seems troubled, I can find out, through writing samples, what is troubling the youngster. You get to the problem more quickly than through psychological tests.

"Two years ago I worked with a child who was out of sphere—in a dreamworld. I analyzed his handwriting, learned what his problems were—trouble in the home. By working with the parents, in two months the child started blossoming and doing good work. When you see a child's problems, and through encouragement, love and understanding, help that child to blossom out—that's the greatest joy."

Although handwriting analysis was just getting underway in Kansas when this interview took place, she predicted its rapid acceptance in other schools, pointing out that it is used extensively in Illinois schools, and is becoming more important in the work of counselors.

IN TEXAS SCHOOLS

Graphoanalysis as a tool for revealing character was introduced into the San Marcos, Texas, school system in the mid-1950s, and its efficacy was attested to by Principal Earl S. Harris who told the *Texas Outlook*: "We tried four years to create a favorable learning attitude in one of our problem children, but not until recently did we find the solution—handwriting analysis. This child came from a good family environment, and was exposed to a well-rounded life. Although he could do well scholastically, he had no desire to attend school. We did everything we could think of, without success.

"Then a graphoanalysis report was secured and among the

traits reported was excellent organizational ability. This trait, coupled with an expressive emotional nature, pointed to one type of leader. The child was given assignments and permitted to share in group responsibilities. Amazingly, he became eager to attend school, and eventually fitted into nearly every phase of the school program. Interestingly, the youngster's neighbors complimented me on the child's new attitude, and it can be categorically stated that this change for the better can be positively traced to the time we received the handwriting analysis. . . ."

Sam Johnson, author of this story, observed: "The puzzling aspects of any particular child's personality can be quickly and accurately determined from the handwriting. . . . The quirks then can be diplomatically sidestepped, or a remedy attempted—but *learning the cause* is the primary step toward cure."

Kenneth D. Farnham of the American Institute of Graphoanalysis says that after the age of eight—when a child has reached the point where attention centers upon the meaning of what is being written rather than the muscular dexterity required— graphoanalysis becomes valuable in character and vocational analysis.

SCRIBBLES HAVE MEANING

Graphoanalyst Robert Wasserman says that even in the scribble stage, children's personalities are revealed to the trained interpreter.

Children usually scribble between the ages of two and six—starting as soon as they can hold a pencil or crayon," he told *The National Enquirer* (November 11, 1975). "The strokes and lines a child makes may look like nothing at all, but if examined carefully, you can learn much about attitudes, emotions, character traits.

"As a child develops, so do his scribblings, and the changes reveal new habits and traits. After age six, the doodles usually are replaced by line drawings.

"If parents will compare my chart to their youngsters' scribbling, they can learn a lot about their habits and personalities. Here are some examples:

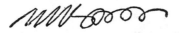

This is a lively, bouncy scribble, showing a spirited child always raring to go.

This slowly made scribble reveals thoughtfulness, sometimes cautiousness, in your child.

The quality and quantity of the line formation here shows us the child is impulsive, changes his mind easily.

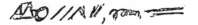

The neatness of this scribble shows a very organized child who will develop good handwriting once the doodling stage is over.

These angular, firm strokes show the child is strong-willed, has a powerful personality.

Roundlike formations of any type tell us the child tends to be kindly, likeable, friendly.

Light pressure or light writing, as in this scribble, discloses a sensitive child with artistic nature.

Heavy pressure, as in this scribble, reveals a firm child who knows what he wants.

Extremely small formations such as those in this scribble show a child with a precise mind who pays attention to detail.

THE SQUIGGLES TELL SO MUCH!

The child: "A masterpiece of a magnificent Creator, destined in all eternity to be happy."

This is a quote from Mother M. Cecilia Koehler of Paola, Kansas, who has specialized for years in teaching a basic graphoanalysis course to nuns for use in coping with children's emotional problems. That subject was discussed during a panel which included Mother Cecilia; Elvira Behrens of Arlington Heights, Illinois; Emilie Stockholm of Chicago who spent many years in counseling and guidance work with preschool and retarded children; and Ruth "Pat" Gough of Buffalo, New York, a teacher of graphoanalysis to parents and teachers.

"To give emotionally disturbed little ones proper guidance," says Mother Cecilia, "we need to understand the child as an individual. We need to realize that this small bit of humanity is endowed with intellect, a free will, and a personality different from any other human being who ever lived, is living today, and who will live in the future.

"So I beg you, be patient and generous with boys and girls...you are dealing with soulstuff. The unique and complex personality of the child has been influenced by heredity, by the environment into which the child was born, and to some extent by the child's free will. These three forces are at work constantly in a child's personality, and their effects produce many and various traits and behavior patterns. Many of these effects are hard to understand and interpret.

"However, as graphoanalysts we realize fully that we have the keys to the personality of the child. We possess the master key to the child's world. When we pick up the handwriting or perhaps the very first scribbles of the child, we can see that powerful forces already have been working on this embryonic character...."

Mother Cecilia introduced Elvira Behrens, a specialist in work with preschool and retarded children. What she had to say may be of interest to people who have already or who are about to take on the responsibilities of parenthood.

Ms. Behrens has accumulated specimens from children who had not yet learned to speak, pre-verbal youngsters. She prefers to call the graphics of these tots "squiggles—spontaneous strokes completely directed by the brain."

The strokes are "less restricted than writing, and reveal more of the uninhibited traits of a child," she maintains. "When a child first learns to write, she concentrates on mechanical execution of the stroke. Squiggles are the undisciplined strokes or gestures of the brain."

This teacher has studied hundreds of squiggles, and while watching the children as they scribbled, found that those under three write in reverse—from right to left. At age three—with exceptional children a few months earlier—Ms. Behrens learned that the child writes in two directions, some strokes forward, some backward, and at this age starts writing "in circles." The squiggles are forward.

"We were taught by Dr. Bunker," she said, "that strokes made in reverse are back to self, reveal thinking to self or living within self. Psychology teaches that children are self-centered, think within self the first few years of life, then come to realize that one must *give* love as well as receive it."

The specialist then displayed squiggles of children starting at nine months. "This specimen," she continued, "is that of a nine-month-old child. Strokes are in reverse, starting at the right, moving to the left. The child is thinking within self. Notice the tapering qualities of the strokes. Some are rather blunt. Under a magnifying glass you can see that they taper to a fine edge which can't be seen with the naked eye. This is rather natural for a child this age—he lets mother and daddy make the decisions.

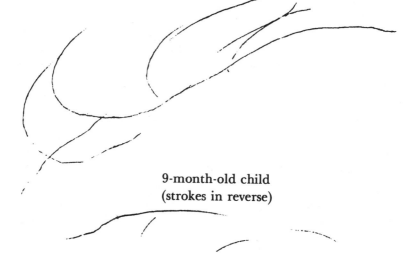

9-month-old child
(strokes in reverse)

"The squiggles below were made by an 18-month-old child. Again, everything is in reverse. Notice in the first specimen, there was nothing whatsoever in the thinking area. In the second specimen, however, before he went up, he made a v-stroke at the bottom. This reveals analytical ability. The upstroke is a far forward slant. It shows a child's emotions. This child is very affectionate. Then at the top is the inquisitive or exploratory point. Note the strong, very long downstroke, showing determination. This child now is beginning to have a desire to learn. In the first year, there is none of this.

18-month-old child
(strokes still in reverse)

"In the next specimen, notice all the irritability jabs—made in reverse. When I saw this I hoped graphoanalysis was wrong, I didn't want to believe there could possibly be that much irritability in the soul of a little baby. However, that day I saw every single one of those irritability jabs in action. It nearly broke my heart.

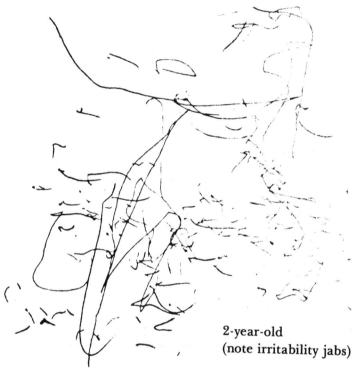

2-year-old
(note irritability jabs)

"Next we see the squiggles of a 3½-year-old child. Notice the investigative interest, the desire to learn, and the pinpoint penetration of thinking which occurs in much of this boy's writing. Strokes show a high degree of analytical thinking, investigation. Here we see the start of the circle strokes—some made forward, others in reverse. If the first line in this specimen were written forward, you would notice the upstroke. Thus it is important in analyzing a child's scribble that you know *which way the child scribbled.* However, this line was written in reverse, so it becomes a downstroke. Since emotions are shown *only in the upstroke,* it is important to know which is which. It changes the emotional pattern completely.

"I told the mother this child was highly inquisitive, that he wanted to learn, asked many questions and insisted on a full answer. She confirmed my findings by telling how he had to learn the hard way that a door closing on a finger will hurt the finger!

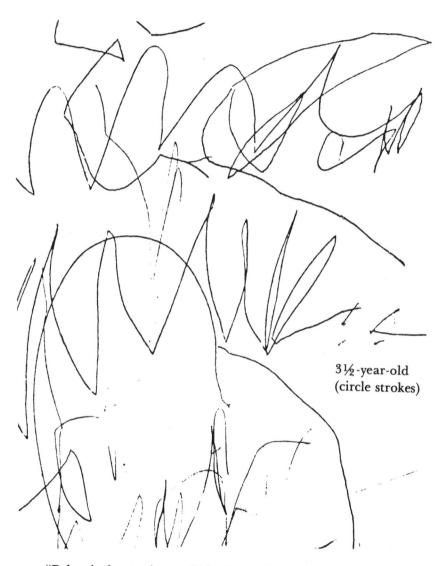

3½-year-old
(circle strokes)

"Below is the specimen of big sister. She's just as affectionate as the little boy. Notice the upstroke—far forward. And the pinpoint penetration of thinking. The broad top strokes and pinpoints show ability to create and do things with her hands. There are many *e*-strokes here—the Greek *e*'s, indicating cultural tendencies. This girl is brilliant. And diplomacy is one of her outstanding traits.

"I have many of her squiggles, all show strokes which taper off to a fine point. When she learned to write, she did this same thing. Always she starts the first letter extremely large, tapering off to letters about half that size. She was only four when I got this squiggle.

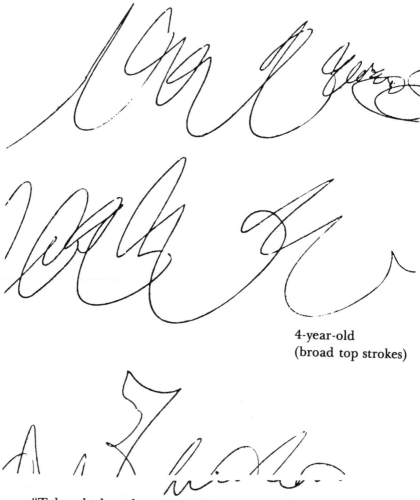

4-year-old
(broad top strokes)

"Take a look at the next specimen. Isn't that beautiful! I say it's beautiful because most people think squiggles are to be tossed into a wastebasket. To me this is beautiful because I see character, personality, emotions. I see affection.

"Notice the extreme pinpoint penetration of thinking here. She was five when this was written. I find more in squiggles than in writing because I analyzed this child's writing at the age of eight, and it showed nearly all rounded tops—not because she is a slow thinker, but she was taught to make rounded tops and conforms to the rules.

"These tops, rounded and so broad, indicate tremendous ability to work with the hands. These should be compared to the broad-topped *r*'s. Look for determination in this kind of writing, and investigative urge. Notice also the secretiveness of the circular letters—she is developing a large measure of that trait.

5-year-old
(pinpoint penetration)

"In the specimen below we have the squiggle of a creative six-year-old boy. Notice all the creative strokes. He sits by the hour, working on something. He is not always a slow thinker, either—there's pinpoint penetration here. A keen mind is developing.

6-year-old
(full of creativity)

"The final specimen belongs to a nine-year-old boy who left an orphanage in Germany for a home in America—and loving foster parents. Note the affection here. But also note the back-slant. This little lad was in the orphanage several years before adoption, and I believe this accounts for his changeable emotions. He has periods of withdrawal—doesn't believe everyone accepts him, and likewise can't bring himself to accept everyone. So he holds back. Oh, he shows his affection readily, but there is a certain amount of withdrawal, too.

"The big loops reveal acquisitiveness. I told the mother this little fellow was content to sit down with a catalog and get excited about what he found. But he also wanted these things. She agreed.

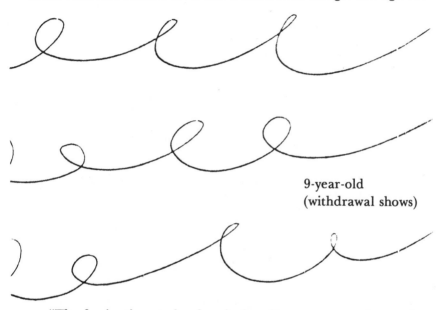

9-year-old
(withdrawal shows)

"The fascinating study of squiggles allows you to understand a child at an early age. These squiggles are made by God's precious children, and they need to be understood."

Mother Cecilia concluded with these comments: "The home into which the child is born is the most important part of the child's world. There is where personality is shaped, the character formed for life. As graphoanalysts, we see these home influences in strokes of writing. In the handwriting of many children we find the reflection of a happy, well-integrated home life, and we appreciate that. However, as analysts, we are more interested in spotting and helping the child with a problem."

Perhaps the most comprehensive research in analysis of children's scribbles was done in the 1930s when the Hungarian government sponsored an eight-year handwriting study in Budapest. More than 2,000 students, 10 to 18 years old, were tested. Most were checked twice a year. Several hundred abnormal children, including stutterers, deaf-mutes, and those exhibiting antisocial behavior were studied for comparison. The late Klara Roman, founder of Budapest's Institute for Psychology of Handwriting, was involved in much of that research. She is another "big name" in the field, taught graphology as a psychological method for the study of personality at the New School for Social Research, New York, and authored the classic *Handwriting: a Key to Personality*, and *Encyclopedia of the Written Word—A Lexicon for Graphology and Other Aspects of Writing*.

THERE'S HELP FOR LEARNING DISABILITY

If your child is among the one in seven in the nation unfortunate enough to have been born with a learning disability (L.D.) making it difficult to read—letters may be upside down or transposed—or to do numbers, or has trouble with body coordination—don't despair. There is help.

The medical term for this disorder is "dyslexia" from the Greek root *dys*, "difficulty," and *lexia*, "pertaining to words." Identified by British and German ophthalmologists in the 19th century, the trouble lies with a slight dysfunction of the brain, resulting in failure to properly decode language symbols.

Not that it's any consolation, but some of the world's greats are believed to have been victims of the baffling ailment: Albert Einstein, Thomas Edison, General George S. Patton, President Woodrow Wilson, Hans Christian Andersen. One of the factors can be an extremely high I.Q. Vice-President Nelson Rockefeller is another who throughout his life has seen "numbers and letters backwards, or think of them backwards." He never mastered spelling, yet graduated cum laude from Dartmouth College and earned a Phi Beta Kappa key. The *Washington Star* carried a story by science and medicine writer Warren R. Young, reproducing from his diary when he was eleven these lines: 'Lunc,' 'picknick Lunch,' 'Uncil Harold,' 'engen repar schop,' 'Parak' [for park]," and three tries at recording the disease his sister Abby had come down with—"'mealess,' 'measless,' and 'misless.'

There is a marvelous new book on the subject of dyslexia from the points of view of those who have had to "overcome" it—it especially tackles the problem of hereditary dyslexia. (Elizabeth Fleming, the author, and all five of her children—all dyslexics—are direct descendants of Woodrow Wilson.) The book is entitled *Believe The Heart: Our Dyslexic Days.*

Studies have shown that 80% of learning disabilities can be corrected if diagnosed and treated before the child enters third grade. The rate drops to half—40%—if L.D. is not diagnosed until fifth-grade age. And if treatment is not started before reaching seventh grade, the chance of remediation is a tragic 5%.

There are four categories of learning disabilities:

Acalculia presents problems in processing numbers.

Dysgraphia is the medical term for lack of muscular coordination in writing.

Aphasia prevents a child from understanding language structure—forming sentences and paragraphs.

Dyslexia—visual or auditory—is the most common form of L.D. and affects the ability to learn language symbols.

Children with auditory dyslexia are confronted with the same problems with the spoken, rather than written, word. Even the most clearly pronounced words reach the brain in a distorted fashion.

Dyslexic children often are afflicted with accompanying related disorders. They may lack a sense of time, of sequence and order, or direction. They cannot freely run and jump because they feel physically disoriented. They may not be able to distinguish left from right. They don't know what comes before or after something. Memories are garbled timewise.

Most L.D. children suffer not only from a combination of sensory and motor difficulties, but may also be hyperkinetic—nervous, jittery, with short attention span.

Hyperkinesis can be relieved. Dr. Ben Feingold of San Francisco has done important work revealing a relationship between this disorder and allergy to food additives. But treatment of learning disabilities is not that easy. At the moment, special schooling for L.D. children is limited, with training concentrated mainly among elementary school children. Ideally, the L.D. child is placed in the controlled environment of a special small class. Here there is training to develop the senses and motor functions least affected by L.D. These children learn to combine the defective functions with the more developed ones. Special exercises are aimed at improving the deficiencies.

KNOW YOUR CHILD

"The way a child writes," wrote the late Antonia Klekoda, an authority in the field for many years, "can warn the parents of possible emotional distress. It reveals conflicts, development, and potential."

This graphologist observed that "nice" handwriting does not necessarily indicate a "nice" character—"it may merely reflect a child's ability to copy the teacher's letter formations as demonstrated on the blackboard.

"A child's physical well-being is displayed, even in penmanship. Pressure is firm and without variance in a normal child's script. Thus:

I have a cat na tabby and a dog. ginger. They sleep t

"Undistorted spacing between letters indicates balance in the child's priorities."

Size, slant, pressure, and spacing are the factors reflecting emotional makeup, Ms. Klekoda continued, listing the following as elements "to be on the lookout for in your child's handwriting:

SIZE

"A beginning writer just naturally writes large in the process of learning letter formation—it does not mean the child is a showoff. If the writing continues large long after completion of the penmanship course, it's a signal that continuing attention is required, not only in the writing but in other areas. That youngster won't take 'no' for an answer, incidentally.

"Handwriting which is neither too large nor too small signifies ability to adjust. And if there's a combination of large and small letter formations in a single sample, it means the child is discovering new identity. As long as irregularity occurs in script size, the youngster is experiencing mixed attitudes, and life poses problems resulting in confrontations."

SLANT

"Handwriting is either upright, bent rightward, or written backhand.

"*Upright* or perpendicular letters belong to a conscientious child, one who checks emotions and exhibits poise. This youngster—boy or girl—is dependable, not prone to display innermost feelings. A logical approach to a situation induces his support and involvement. Children with vertical writing show concern for their responsibilities.

"*Right leaning* handwriting is a clue to an affectionate individual—if the tilt is 45 degrees, gregariousness is a more descriptive word.

"Friendship is important to the writer whose letters are slanted. But beware if the slant rightward becomes too extreme—give that child definite responsibilities and make certain they are carried out. Too much slant reveals a trend to moodiness.

"*Backhand* writing conveys the message of a reserve personality. It suggests the more secretive child, cautious about personal commitment to others."

PRESSURE

"Heavy writing is an expression of deep feelings. The darker the imprint, the more impressionable the child. Life is meaningful for this youngster, relationships are sincere.

"Developing impulses and strong driving forces are nourished in the child with heavy-pressured script. Situations may inflate out of perspective, and this writer will stew over letdowns, be rapturous with success, and occasionally experience seemingly infinite frustrations.

"Light-pressured handwriting reveals personality with short-lived, somewhat delicate impressions. This child is not apt to be a braggart or the pushy type. Often he is indifferent."

SPACING

"Pinched handwriting indicates selfishness—either with personal belongings, enthusiasms, or talents. This child should be encouraged toward group participation.

"Sprawled, wide-spaced handwriting suggests expensive whims, an impractical nature. Unrealistic pursuits, and parental yielding to extravagant demands almost certainly will develop into wasteful habits. The child will be fortunate in later life if taught a respect for money."

FURTHER CHECKLIST

"Repeated spelling errors in simple words are a signal the youngster is not concentrating.

"Short endings are a clue to an abrupt disposition that frequently makes it difficult for the child to pursue a pleasant association with peers.

"A hesitant child dots the *i* to the left of the letter, and the *t* does not cross through the stem.

"Tight strokes at the beginning of a letter will tell the analyst that the youngster is defensive and lacks confidence.

"Ornamental writing reveals feelings of inadequacy. Feeling overlooked, this child may create a fuss to gain attention, behavior becoming obnoxious at times.

"Confused style indicates a confused writer. Character defects such as deceit—lying—are revealed if the *i* is not dotted, the *t* is not crossed, and letter formation is careless.

"A self-controlled, cooperative nature shows in a combination of angular and round writing.

"Handwriting is a reliable guide to a child's potential, and at the same time reveals the characteristics which can inhibit realization of that potential, or make it a reality.

"The parent who will take the time to learn the basics of

handwriting analysis can apply the knowledge to the child's everlasting benefit. By observing changes in the writing, the parent is alerted to personality changes. The knowledgeable parent thus has a valid tool for understanding the youngster's physical, mental, and spiritual needs."

DON'T TEACH CONFORMISM!

"Outdated" penmanship teaching methods retard mental and emotional development of many youngsters, says Mrs. Beryl Hamilton, Tucson, Arizona, a teacher for 30 years, a former vice-president of the American Association of Handwriting Analysts.

"Forcing a child to sit in a prescribed position and write in a prescribed way can cause frustration," she believes. "Such methods can cause character breakdown, particularly in a sensitive child, and create emotional disturbances that may last a lifetime. I am convinced that many delinquents actually are a result of forced, unreal penmanship lessons.

"Teachers in grade schools expect students to write with perfect, rounded, flowing letters. Students are told how to hold a pencil, how to hold the paper at the correct angle, how to sit erect, how to place their feet."

These positions, she said, "usually are abandoned for their own individual style because they know instinctively what is best and most comfortable for themselves.

"Rather than trying to stifle individual style, teachers should strive only to make sure students can write legibly. After all, the purpose of writing is communication, not little 'cookie-cutter,' rubber-stamp examples of conformity."

She suggests students be encouraged to write with either or both hands in a "normal, natural style, with a maximum of simplicity."

(Editor's note: A valuable method of increasing mental acuity.)

This point of view is shared by Dr. Anthony Becker, Elgin, Illinois, psychologist, a former president of A.A.H.A.: "Emotional problems in children relate to repressions in classrooms where teachers insist on too much adherence to copybook style of handwriting, unnatural to the child's personality."

LaMont McConnell, special education administrator in Tucson, concurs: "Handwriting reflects personality, and when a student is forced into a specific handwriting mold it can harm personality. Making rounded, perfect, flowing letters slows down the thought process."

The ABCs of
Handwriting Analysis

Handwriting analysis is performed by reducing script to its basic elements, analyzing the pieces, and interpreting the whole.

Basic features include:

(1) Form

　　(Size)

(2) Movement

　　(Pressure)

These are further reduced to such elements as:

(a) Change of margin

(b) Slant

(c) Height and width of letters

(d) Spacing between letters, and words, and other characteristics.

"Any exaggeration in a script—be it pressure, size, slant, or other features, is looked upon as a gesture toward compensation or overcompensation of some deficiency," said the late Alfred G. Mendel in *Personality in Handwriting*.

Since we write to communicate, *illegibility is assumed as an avoidance of communication*. Exaggeration may mean anything from conceit and arrogance to neurotic anxiety and secretiveness. *Words* are symbols by which we communicate, either by talking, or writing. *Form* also is a language—did you ever think of it thus?

Form, size, movement, pressure, reveal aspects of the "inner self"—personality—projected on paper through handwriting, which as William Preyer said three quarters of a century ago, actually is "brainwriting." Whether the pencil or pen is held by teeth, toes (as with some polio victims and others), or by fingers, the writer unwittingly produces a self-portrait. Our writing is a recording of our will, urges, emotions.

HIGH FORM LEVEL: The handwriting of the person possessing the positive traits of naturalness, originality, order, rhythm, balance, firmness:

LOW FORM LEVEL: Handwriting which reflects the absence of positive traits, revealing instead such negative characteristics as instability and confused outlook. Graphic signs of this personality are uneven margins, distorted letter shapes, erratically spaced letters and words, a rising and falling base line.

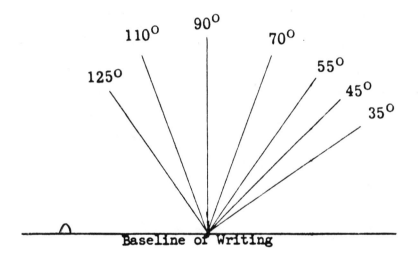

Clues to your social and emotional inclinations are revealed in the slant of your writing:

From an art or stationery store, get yourself a protractor, an instrument for laying down and measuring angles—preferably one with a closed center. Under a specimen of your handwriting, using a sharp pencil, lightly draw the base line, touching as many letters as possible, and using care not to ruin the specimen. As in the sample below, individual words may require separate base lines. Then place straight edge of protractor along base line, with center-point of protractor on the stroke being measured. Read slant angle indicated on protractor. Words falling below or rising above the total line of writing should be measured in accordance with their own base line, as below.

Sample:

RIGHT SLANT: If your handwriting slants to the right, you
have a lively interest in the future, and tendencies toward social
and extrovertive behavior—you like people, and want to keep
moving ahead.

LEFT SLANT: Leftward movement (backhand) in handwriting implies emphasis on the past—regression, if you want to call it that. This personality tends to be introverted. Antisocial tendencies may be measured by the degree of the slant leftward. This trait could be a result of repressed childhood experiences. The person whose writing takes such a slant possesses a certain degree of reserve, caution, and fear of the future. Left slant also can indicate a talented homemaker who enjoys solitude. Such an individual favors the traditional pattern, is oriented to the past.

VERTICAL SLANT: If you form letters vertically, you live in the present, and your decisions are based on reason rather than emotion—you're ruled by your head, not your heart. You have a measure of reserve, lack of spontaneity, and acquaintances find you self-controlled, self-reliant.

appreciate your trouble.

test procedures
trouble shooting
with machines,
re characteristics

(Finance Dept.) is coming back
Venezuela in April + I plan
meet him in Mexico — but
like we're all going to wind up
back in Great Falls before
long — ugh!

From some fool he
Who wanted me
To be his ...

Thank you very much for your accurate .
exactly what my weaknesses are and I will endea...
them, while I am making a study of graphol...
to be subjective — and hence I did not care to .
· ...jective element is subtle, you know, ...

g through your bo
and I find it all
...ave had friends w
...ery enlightening re

To banish this negative, hurtful personality trait, do this exercise:

the this at

DECISIVENESS

The decisive person is able to make a firm choice between possible courses of action without vacillating. This trait—a "healthy" one—is identified by strong ending strokes of words:

The decisive person will never evade facing a problem

Indecisiveness—vacillation—reveals itself when word-endings are written thus:

indecisive person will bring the last letter a firm finish

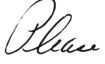
Please Excuse this informal

My father passed months ago and, after

VARIABLE SLANT: This characteristic in handwriting denotes an individual apt to plunge impulsively ahead on one occasion, and retreat without warning into a state of judgment and poise on another—erratic behavior. This is the guy or gal you never quite know how to gauge. Play a harmless joke on him—one that would amuse him today—he might respond with irritation or outright anger tomorrow. These unpredictable reactions can't help but affect relationships with others, who understandably eventually find it difficult to maintain a comfortable relationship with such a person.

Your emotional response to your social environment is plainly visible to the analyst through the slant of letter formations: if *rightward*, you are emotionally free to move ahead with projects and life generally; the *vertical* slant shows that you control reactions; and *backhand* slant confirms that you prefer the past, or traditional, repressing forward movement.

You may choose to meet environment easily (FORWARD SLANT).

I am very interested
in handwriting analysis
and curious to know what

Or you may resist (BACKWARD SLANT).

do ? I thought up to this

Percusionist, spoons, traps
sculls etc etc.
live in the country jus'
itside of London.

Backhand writing indicates withdrawal. This individual is inclined to evaluate consequences before committing herself. A consistent, moderate slant manifests control and balance.

RELATIONSHIPS

Each of us moves *toward*, or *away* from people, depending on our emotional needs. This movement is related to the shape of the letters in our handwriting.

Letters are formed by *curved* (flexible)

Enclosed is the check for the lesson material Jack picked up.

or *straight* (inflexible) strokes.

silently minding

Strokes indicate one's emotional needs in relating to others. Where do you fit — are your relationships essentially flexible, yielding?

Strokes indicating the relationship areas are the connecting forms that join letters. Usually they're found in the middle zone, and are called *garlands*, *angles*, and *arcades*.

Garland: The garland is easy to execute, requiring minimum effort. The ease and speed of execution produces a harmonious effect. The curves and blending qualities, and the bowl form, symbolize openness to influence from the nonmaterial sphere. It can be in the spiritual, emotional, social, and action areas. The garland indicates adaptability, sociability, attitudes toward the future, flexibility — capacity to adjust to others — and is a balancing and blending quality. The form level determines whether the garland originates within the context of positive or negative attitudes. If negative, it can mean the individual avoids decisions, may be too easily influenced by others, and resists facing the future — reality. Positive:

rau into 90 minutes

Angle: The angle indicates rigidity, resistance to environmental influences. The analytical and exploratory personality uses this form of connecting letters. Such a writer is technically inclined, exact and precise in thought-processes. Nothing is taken for granted, it's got to be personally investigated.

I hope it will reach you safely and in go
Please drop me a line to say the print has
good order.

Arcade: The arcade is the joining stroke at the top of letters. It may appear as an arch, as the name implies. Arcades are viewed by the analyst as the element of constructability — the writer forms conclusions, deliberately builds ideas or objects step-by-step, methodically adding layer atop layer. The arcade is open at the bottom, the arch protecting the writer from the outside world and from at least some of the influences from emotional and social relationships. Arcades in writing are interpreted as indicating reserve, secrecy in the writer.

I am only too happy to send
you a specimen of my stylized handwriting, which is a variant of the old

OUTWITTING TOMORROW; WRITTEN DOWN BY FRATER VIII

Outwitting Tomorrow is especially intended for men and women in all walks of life who are striving to attain individuality. By knowing and practicing a few simple rules and secrets, and by doing what you can, with what you have, wherever you are *now*, it is possible to bring about results and changes in your life and affairs that may astound you, regardless of your age, education, health, environment, or financial circumstances.

Throughout the lifetime of man upon this earth, his actions and thoughts fall into five separate and distinct divisions or departments. His success in living depends entirely upon how well he has expanded and used these five departments of life. A star ably represents them; each point indicating a particular department. The uppermost point represents the spiritual; the upper right one, the mental; the upper left, the physical; the lower right one is the social; and the lower left, the financial. These five divisions completely cover every phase of an individual's life, regardless of what diverse names they bear. They remain unalterable, constant, and resistantly fixed.

Life holds but one purpose. A purpose which is inexorably decreed by destiny; that each human being, starting from the center of his individual star, must fill out the departments of life represented by the points, evenly and symmetrically, taking care that one point be not greatly developed beyond the others, but rather that they be expanded alike.

Herewith are five stars. Each one shows a particular department of life over-developed at the expense of the other four. This is what occurs when one does not have clearly in mind the fact that there are five deparments of life. Lacking that knowledge, it is impossible to develop, enlarge, and expand all *five* evenly and symmetrically; one is always bound to be eccentric and abnormal. Is it any wonder, then, that the average person experiences so much sorrow, ill-health, fear, and poverty?

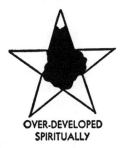

**OVER-DEVELOPED
SPIRITUALLY**

Over-developed spiritually

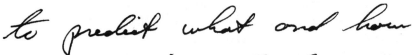

The first star of the series shows a person who is over-developed spiritually or religiously. He is "all heart and no head." Except along very narrow and bigoted lines, reason, will, and judgment are warped and stunted. Although called a spiritual or religious type, very often this person's beliefs are so narrow and intolerant that he really isn't spiritual at all, merely fanatical. His friends are of like character, and because he imagines them to be more religious than himself, he becomes jealous of their activities; thus he is usually anti-social. Physically, this person is only a fraction of what he could be. He is inclined to dyspepsia, anemia, and nervous disorders. He possesses little of this world's goods. Not that he wouldn't accept what was offered with the fervor of a miser, but because he is in such an appalling mental state and is so strait-laced and unyielding in his religious practices that he drives everything of an abundant and opulent nature from him.

OVER-DEVELOPED
MENTALLY

Over-developed mentally

MASTER INC., AS PLA.
THE LAST SIX (6) MON
EXPERIENCE HAS BEEN
AND ENGINEERING IN

With the help of my parents,
the Langley Porter Clinic for 7 we
ly recovered and was able to func
being with the aid of tranquilize

The second star represents a person who is over-developed in the mental department of life. He lacks spirituality; reasoning that if God cannot be found between the covers of a book or in a test tube then most certainly there is no God. Like the spiritually over-developed, he is narrow, bigoted, and intolerant of those who do not share his opinions. Caring little for physical exertion, his health is usually in a deplorable state; while socially, he confines himself to associates of the same mental turn as himself. Living constantly in theory, he is highly impractical, and only by the greatest effort can he manage to support himself comfortably.

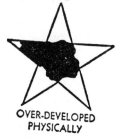

OVER-DEVELOPED
PHYSICALLY

Over-developed physically

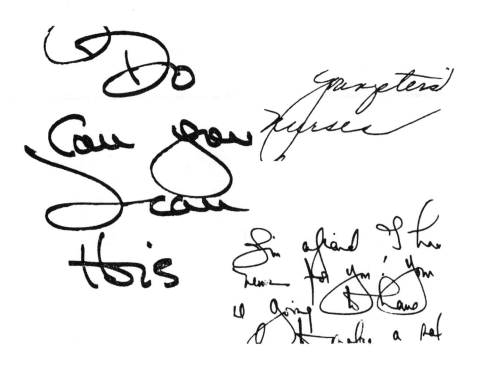

The physically over-developed is shown by the third star. Strong and robust, he is the typical male animal, noisy and domineering. The spiritual side of his nature has never developed; but this much can be said to his credit: He seldom denies the existence of that which he doesn't understand or in which he has little interest. He is below average mentally, running more to muscle than to mind. Socially, he is popular with that class of people who see beauty in the movements of bulging muscles. He is usually in modest financial circumstances due to the fact that through physical effort he is capable of earning enough money to satisfy the wants of his physical nature; so he does not concern himself about accumulating wealth until his earning capacity begins to fail him.

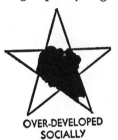

OVER-DEVELOPED
SOCIALLY

Over-developed socially

The fourth star typifies the individual who is over-developed in the social department of life. He is of the hail-fellow-well-met variety. An innocuous hand-shaker who, due to his affable nature, comes by many free meals and alcoholic drinks. Spiritually, mentally, physically, and financially he is in pretty poor shape; having neglected them all in favor of being sociable. Occasionally he falls into a remunerative political job, or is retained as a professional greeter, but as a rule he leads a hand-to-mouth existence.

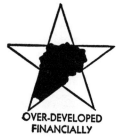

OVER-DEVELOPED
FINANCIALLY

Over-developed financially

your book and.

nclosed on a separate
ny writing and the.
/by you in your le.

handwriting and.

My shame is doubled, first by having
srrow'd now by being so late in the
- of your loan— I assure you that
heque is not made of gutta purcha!

The financial department of life is shown over-developed by the fifth star. This type of person might very reasonably have been an all-around, evenly-developed individual before the mania for money struck him. He has the ability to fill out the other four points of his star, but once having succumbed to the craving for wealth he rapidly becomes stunted and dwarfed in everything else. He goes to his grave with an insatiable desire for more and still more wealth, and fears and abhors death because it deprives him of his material gain. Usually he is devoid of friends, and has sacrificed his spiritual heritage in his lust for money. His health is rarely good because of neglect, and his mentality is limited in scope to schemes for more wealth and power.

These five stars show the extremes in over-development of one particular department of life, but it's seldom that any one is of such an exceptionally eccentric type. Usually it is a variation or combination of these types. Often two points are emphasized; in some three, and less often four are well-developed. However, there is always one point which is woefully neglected, and which retards progress in the other four. Destiny dares not permit an individual to become too highly developed in four departments of life without developing the fifth. Such a being would become a colossal menace to society, especially if the spiritual department was the dwarfed point of his star.

Hoping to receive the
nal Certificate I am,
Sincerely,

(Finance Dept.) is coming back
Venezuela in April + I plan
meet him in Mexico — But
like we're all going to wind u
back in Great Falls before
long — ugh!

Now we come to the star which indicates an even, equal, steady development in all five departments of life. This person gives little promise at first of being in any way exceptional. But as he fills out his star he becomes powerful and power-filled. He starts accomplishing things, and his accomplishments are real and lasting, for he has built on a symmetrical foundation which is solid and strong. Results are noticeable to everyone when this individual has even half-filled in all points; from then on he will completely fill in the entire star in a very short time and become a competent, all-around super-individual. He is in harmony with all that is constructive in both the visible and unseen worlds. Forces which would frighten the ordinary, eccentrically-developed person into convulsions, are his friends and allies. They race to do his bidding.

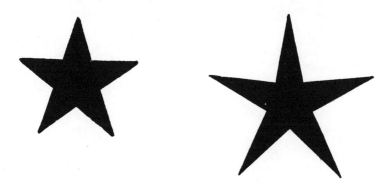

But this is not the end. There is no end. Once a star has been completely filled in there are still greater things to strive for. These star points are capable of unlimited extension and can continually be pushed out into added achievements in all five departments of life. This process of extension is shown by the last star with the elongated points. There is no limit to the length of these points. Long points become longer ones as the individual marches onward in his conquests. And when one has experienced thrilling *expansion* in all five departments of life, there is no turning back. From then on it's a search for "more worlds to conquer."

To he who by this humble discourse, and its still more humble illustrations, manages to "catch fire" in his quest for *expansion* in the five departments of life, there are no limits, no sorrows, no more darkness. From then on all is bright, joyous, radiant and thrilling.

PHYSIOLOGICAL AFFLICTIONS AND THEIR PSYCHO-LOGICAL ORIGIN

Of the hundreds of physical afflictions to which the flesh is heir, there are but two causes. The first is of a strictly physiological origin; the second is of a psychological origin. Of the two, the psychological is said to be by far the more prevalent.

Herewith is a short list of physical afflictions and their psychological causes. As you may note, many of these afflictions have more than one cause.

Apoplexy—Brought on by anger, hate or extreme passion.
Back lameness—Burden-bearing thoughts.
Biliousness—Revengeful, traitorous, mutinous thoughts.
Boils and other eruptions—Irritability, impatience.
Catarrh—Disgust, disdain, and false superiority.
Cancer—Dissatisfied love nature, selfishness, frustration.
Colds—Depressions, despondency, "the blues."
Constipation—Nervous tension, worry, lack of poise.
Croup—Intense irritation and confusion.
Deafness—Unwillingness to listen, judge, and accept.
Diarrhea—Tendency to run away or avoid reality.
Diphtheria—Intensified resistance to truth and reality.
Goiter—Obstinate pride, fear of difficulties.
Hay fever—lack of interest, self-inflicted limitations.
Headache—Confusion, fear, worry, brain exhaustion.
Heart trouble—Selfishness, fear, worry, tension.
Hemorrhoids—Prolonged anxiety, fear, and worry.
Hysteria—Repression, mental conflicts, selfishness.
Kidney trouble—Inferiority complex, fear of detection.
Liver trouble—Inaction, depression, repression.
Nausea—Rejection of facts or truth, emotional conflicts.
Paralysis—Thwarted or inhibited desires.
Pneumonia—Overwhelming disappointment of long duration.
Rheumatism—Fault-finding, criticism, nagging.
Sore throat—Unconscious resistance to truth.
Spinal trouble—Remote fear of death and eternal judgment.
Stomach trouble—Oversensitiveness, rejection of facts.
Frigidity—(In either sex) Repression, conflicts, shocks.
Tuberculosis—Lack of freedom or a shut-in complex.
Urinary trouble—Inefficiency, inability, and "I can't."

The mental department, like the spiritual, is capable of being grossly misunderstood. Many people confuse intelligence with education. The mental department is divided into three realms: the conscious, the subconscious, and the super-conscious. The sub-conscious takes care of habitual thoughts and actions and consists of memory, imagination, belief, affection, emotion, and conscience. The super-conscious is the realm of the spiritual side of man's nature and works through the sub-conscious, using the qualities of inspiration, intuition, and genius. But about these two realms we are not directly concerned at this time. We are, however, directly concerned with the conscious mind, for here dwell reason, will, and judgment. The development of these three mental qualities marks the difference between education and intelligence; for if these qualities are lacking, education is merely a matter of memory.

An educated man with a highly developed ability to reason and judge, and with a strong will is, of course, invaluable. You seldom find him working for someone else. Then there are comparatively uneducated. people who have a more highly developed reason, will, and judgment than do the college-trained ones, and who are usually found at the head of a great business undertaking or of widespread public projects. So regardless of how limited one's education may be, if he has reason, will, and judgment; if he knows what he wants to do; if he has sufficient zeal, fervor, and enthusiasm, he will succeed in doing great things in spite of the handicaps of age, environment, and circumstance. He will outwit tomorrow.

UPPER ZONE
MIDDLE ZONE
LOWER ZONE

UPPER ZONE is the area of the abstract, intangible, nonphysical—the superconscious. This area gives us a reading on how one thinks, one's goals, extent of the imaginative process, ethical standards, and perception of self-worth. If upper stems are more than three times the height of the middle zone letters, it is a good bet the person is out of touch with reality, certainly does not have his or her "feet on the ground."

If the upper stems are more than three times as high than the middle zone letters

MIDDLE ZONE (mundane) denotes the area over which we have direct control and command, the realm in which we are physically active. This is the graphic area of conscious activity, daily routine, social behavior, relations, and preferences. Handwriting in this zone reveals the visible portion of our personality as seen by acquaintances.

analysis of my handwriting. now I know

run to the utmost of my ability to over

rgy I feared that my analysis would

iddle zone is the area

cious activity, daily

re, social behavior

LOWER ZONE is the storehouse of our experiences and feelings—pleasant and unpleasant. Childhood memories, relationships with parents and friends, as well as the instinctive capacities for pleasure and pain, joy and sorrow, are stored here. Also reflected in the lower zone are material values—those associated with sex, comfort, money, personal values.

The lower zone is the storehouse of our experiences and feelings

If your writing in the upper zone is dwarfed, joined to a large middle zone, it tells the analyst you are too concerned with social relationships at the expense of intellectual and spiritual pursuits.

If your upper zone is dwarfed joind to a large middle zone

Large script in the middle zone, combined with recessed or declining length of letters in the lower zone, means you are too involved with social relationships, not sufficiently concerned with your material requirements and instincts. Your emotional reactions to daily living reflect insecurity because you are inattentive to your own emotional needs, and disregard the need for their expression.

Large script in the middle zone you are too deeply involved with social relationships

Abnormally large middle zone writing also tells us you are overimpressed with your own importance, too deeply engrossed with self, possess little concern for others. We label these traits as part of the immaturity syndrome.

abnormally middle zone tells us you are overimpressed with your own importance

If upper and lower zones are of substantial size, but middle zone is small in comparison, you are not a well-integrated person, unfortunately. You neglect and disregard the need to express emotional response to the stimuli in the day-to-day life experience.

handwriting should be balanced. This indicates a disregard of the need

If your writing shows marked attention in size and elaboration in the lower zone—at the expense of the middle and upper ones—you lack rhythm in the equilibrium. This writing characteristic indicates lack of balance in distribution of your interests, causing you to be short-sighted in judgments.

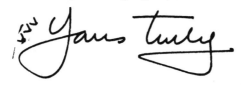

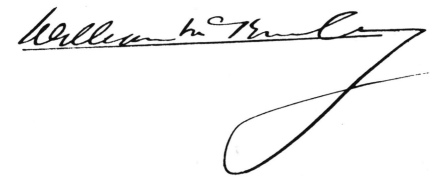

HEAVY PRESSURE

Handwritng expresses the total force uniting our energies, our muscle strength, sex drive, brainpower. It is heavy or light, even or uneven in pressure. Heavy pressure signifies material drive, physical strength, self-confidence, strong sex drive, love of eating, and a dominant, sensuous personality. Firm, strong pressure is indicative of a capacity for visual memory, and firm, even strokes signal manual dexterity. Heavy pressure may imply a stong voice, articulate expression. If you belong in this group, you are serious-minded, have plenty of endurance, and are persistent in work habits. You absorb and retain emotional experiences, and the sum of their effects actually becomes a part of your personality.

LIGHT PRESSURE

Light pressure goes hand-in-hand with reduced drive, occupationally as well as sexually. Check it out—you'll find high sensitivity, timidity. This personality may respond as quickly to emotional stimuli as the heavy-line writer, but the incident is quickly "brushed off"—a trait which the heavy-line writer might label as "fickle."

se the information has of some help to you Many thanks, Jan

Downstrokes showing no pressure, but upstrokes, curves, and lateral strokes made with emphasized pressure, are an indicator of "displaced libido."

Pressure on an upstroke occurs if one perceives environment as hostile; the pressure is a mechanical but subconscious form of resistance. The cause in such cases frequently is pathological, since it is an expression of displaced vitality and possible sensuality.

proper gauge

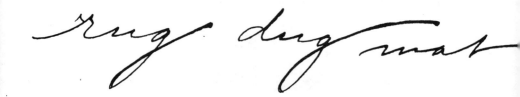

rug dug mat

VARIATIONS

Nervous exhaustion and mental illness may first be exposed in handwriting. Displaced pressure also occurs in the writing of those suffering from arthritis.

Misplaced pressure appears frequently during puberty, an expression of the sudden blocking of the libido (sex urge). Recurrence in later years often means this part of the state of adolescence has not completed its cycle. Inflated pressure occurs during menstruation, pregnancy, menopause, and in the handwriting of persons suffering from gallbladder, kidney, or some heart conditions.

Misplaced emphasis of pressure, as in upstrokes, finals, or embellishments, is a key to a writer's overconcern with nonessentials. When appearing in the initial letter of a word, the introductory gesture implies special caution, perhaps cunning.

Emphasized (heavy pressure) finals show us that communication is emphasized at the last moment with extraordinary force. It tells us that a sense of vitality and willfulness, obstinacy, probably arrogance, are present—particularly when the final stroke is enlarged. This gesture corresponds to a pushing away—rejection—or pronounced expression of reservation.

A forceful, shortened final expresses a command which does not tolerate contradiction!

Pressure in angular forms, decreasing toward the base line, results in needle-like letter-forms—a classical expression of over-sensitivity.

Low pressure invariably indicates sensitivity, often limited to irritability with oneself.

PASTOSITY

"Pastosity" means a stroke uniform in width, dense with ink, outlines blurred. It may suggest sensuous self-indulgence to varying degrees. If pastosity becomes smeary writing—if dots and blotches frequently fill the curvy movements—the picture has changed: If there's only a smattering of this characteristic in the writing, it reveals the sentimentality of a person uncertain of feelings. If the smears are a regular part of writing, it points to fatigue, often the first sign of illness. This characteristic in handwriting appears occasionally after physical or sexual overexertion, and is found in persons suffering from disturbances in the circulatory system. Such "pasty" writing often is combined with interruptions of strokes, due to gallbladder or liver diseases, biliousness, heart ailments.

Smeary writing may appear in cases of hysteria where it is joined by an unclear thread formation, sudden changes in size of letters, and other forms indicating a disturbed balance, and extreme instability.

Pasty writing with relatively weak pressure suggests a personality preoccupied with gratification of the senses, with little activity or interest in other areas.

DIRECTION OF LINES

Does your writing tend to "go uphill" on an unlined page? Yes? Then you're an optimist. You tend to believe things will turn out well. "Ascending writing" also can mean the writer has a compulsion to communicate, and it sometimes occurs during excitement caused by anger.

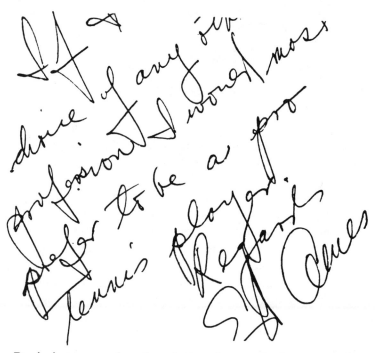

Pessimism can be found in the outlook of one whose handwriting on an unlined page "descends," slopes downward. This characteristic also can signify deep depression, sadness, or fatigue.

Consistently straight-across-the-page writing is that of the person whose emotions are under control, known to acquaintances as the "reliable" type.

LETTERS

If your letters are large, you belong to the category of individuals who "think big," abhor detail, and possess almost unlimited vitality. You think well of yourself, want ample space in which to function, are active, restless.

d like this Deposit
uy Passbook.
Thanks, my new
o-gist Friend.
lots of this writing

Formation of small letters may result from a slight ego impulse. If this characterizes your writing, you are excellent with detail work, have exceptional concentrative ability. Creative persons and scientists often write in small script.

es entschuldigen zu müssen, dass sie dafür waren,
dass man den Tieren Teilnahme erzeigte, wo sie
zugehörig
doch nicht als zu uns gehörig angesehen werden
konnten. Kaum hie und da war in einem der Werke
zu lesen, dass man dem Mitleid und den Tieren
grössere Beachtung als bisher zu schenken habe.

DEGREE OF CONNECTION

If the letters in your writing are always connected, you are logical in your thinking, "sensible." The degree of connection measures the degree to which you've been able to adapt the "I" to "you"—meaning to what extent you have learned to relate to yourself in these aspects: The practical, theoretical, and moral areas of your life.

Unless contradicted by other features of one's handwriting, the person whose letters are routinely connected can be expected to evince the qualities of a practically-, theoretically-, and morally-average character.

College dealing with all Quality. My unit are all - my associate of science

The music was

On the other hand, exaggerated connection—of two or more words, or an entire line—reveals illogical thought-processes. Some people connect words to appear "clever," but actually it spells laziness.

a consisted of more than

BEGINNING AND ENDSTROKES

The beginning strokes of a word reveal, in the variations, the degree of self-reliance and self-esteem we possess. The horizontal space—width—of a letter tells the trained analyst where the writer is positioned on the extroversion-introversion scale. Form and shape of the letter reflect personality.

Handwriting contains the movement from the "I" to the "you." Just as the beginning form of the word tells us something about the writer's character, so does the form of the word ending. The symbol at the end of each word records the writer's current behavior pattern—the present. It represents the qualities related to adaptability (or the opposite) to environment. The word finals (last strokes of words) therefore show one's attitude—formed by past experiences—toward one's fellow man and the world around us.

Aggressive:

affect my day

pock end

Uncommunicative:

Hondwriting

Diplomatic:

streamline writing more

Stubborn:

the amount indicated

Generous, cheerful:

several

groups going

Long initial strokes originating from the left when starting to form words are "tension strokes," stemming from thoughts bound to past experiences (and home environment). Subconsciously we conform to and are dependent upon past instructions. (1)Beginning strokes are taught in early cursive writing, but as writing becomes a more automatic process, we tend to eliminate the initial strokes. If we retain them in adult life, we haven't fully matured. The shorter the inital stroke becomes, the more independence of thought we've acquired. The long inital stroke can be likened to a supporting stick—those who've eliminated it are able to distinguish between important and nonessential issues. (2) Absence of beginning strokes on the letters *a*, *b*, *f*, *h*, *m*, *n*, *o*, *r*, *t*, *u*, *v*, *w*, and *y* indicate direct thinking, the capacity to think and act with speed, to begin without time-consuming preliminaries.

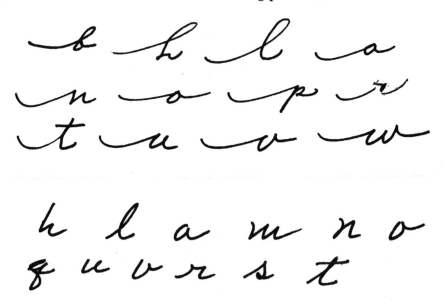

Stiff, rigid, inflexible beginning strokes at or below the base line indicate a defensive nature. This is known as a "resentment" stroke on the circle letters (*a*, *o*, *d*, *g*), and *c*, *m*, *n*, *r*, *u*, *v*, *w*, *y*. It relates to emotions, and a tendency to guard against impositions. When appended to *t*, *h*, or *k*, it is considered a springboard effect and has more to do with abstract thought and attitudes. If the stroke is curved, there is no resentment or resistance.

[handwriting samples: a o d g e]

[handwriting samples: t h k t h]

[handwriting samples: handwriting rawolyn / ly you and saw / free handwriting a / of this very intoves]

Initial strokes formed in a small right circle on lower-case and capital letters, as on *m* and *n*, are evidence that jealousy is focused on one person.

[handwriting samples: m m n n]

Script in which beginning and endstrokes of a word are omitted, discloses a practical nature. This person recognizes essentials, wastes no time or energy on insignificant preliminaries, is not interested in gossip or "small talk."

[handwriting samples: letter is being]

The endstroke of the last letter of a word reveals social attitude. If the last letter is the largest, it can indicate an extremely candid, probably too-outspoken, tactless type of person. It also reveals a person with limited knowledge of human nature, and often appears in the script of adults who haven't grown up.

[handwriting samples: person with limited / knowledge]

A decrease in the size of letters at the end of words reflects diplomacy, sufficient reserve to withhold information if necessary.

decrease in the size of letters indicate diplomacy

Long finals (at least twice as long as the space between letters) disclose generosity.

this year well

(1) An endstroke written with an outburst of pressure indicates aggressive traits — a person unable to control emotions. Sometimes these tensions are released through criminal acts.

(2) Rising (ascending) endstrokes with no emphasis on pressure are signs of aspirations, ambition, an optimistic approach to life, enthusiasm in sharing talents.

writing depth

writing depth

A turned-down endstroke points to a personality unruffled, composed, with matter-of-fact outlook.

a turned down last stroke

If the last stroke of the letter *n* doesn't reach base line, the writer can be expected to conceal facts, is reluctant to acknowledge he has witnessed some incident, and is afraid to expose thoughts. The person with this personality trait also finds it next to impossible to make decisions.

ambition can did it

The initial tick (short, angular stroke preceding the first downward stroke of *m* or *n*) indicates a temper. This has a relationship to the meaning of the letters — *m* indicating interest in problems and illness, *n* in finding and removing obstacles.

New moon middle makes

An endstroke culminating with a small hook demonstrates tenacity. Tenacity hooks elsewhere in the script, on ending strokes, have the same meaning.

an endstroke culminating with a small hook

In lower lengths we find interest in physical activity, material values, sexual urges. Extended underlengths frequently occur in the handwriting of sportsmen and those who use their legs extensively, also those dealing in finance and economics. There is emphasis in the lower zone by the materialist, the realist. Heavy pressure applied to the extended lower lengths indicates material interests based on physical and vital needs. Strong downstrokes reveal a person of strong urges, and determination in carrying through work to completion. Feeble or weak downstrokes reaching into the lower zone often reveal despondency.

Strong in execution:

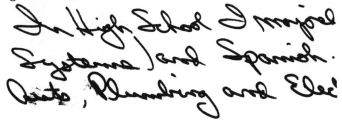

[handwriting sample]

Weak in execution:

[handwriting sample]

SYMMETRY

Symmetry—balanced proportions—is a yardstick of inner balance and development. If the upper zone alone is strongly developed, we are dealing with a person of intelligence and ambition whose emotional development has remained static from childhood, and who has little success fulfilling undertakings.

[handwriting sample]

If upper and middle zones are strongly developed, but not the lower zone, it's an indication the person lacks material orientation and concern—essential in successful planning.

Now that you are

Overdevelopment of one zone invariably occurs at the expense of one or both of the others. The consequence of one-sided excess is lack of inner balance. This makes for deeply dissatisfied, unruly, revolutionary, and "explosive" humans. Symmetry in handwriting (serenity) also is threatened through excessive pressure.

*ly written with letters
However, this pen is per-
y all my writing.*

SPACING

We can immediately recognize and measure the rhythm in space of a handwriting sample by looking at its space pattern—whether in harmony with the spaces between lines, between words, between letters. Disharmony is readily discernible.

*that they can read easily
write at the rate of from,
words per minute and here
How do you like it?*

The space between lines is another feature that can be identified and analyzed at first sight. "Normal" between-lines spacing means you think clearly, interpersonal relationships are realistic, and you are "well-organized"—and a "good organizer."

When spacing between lines is excessively wide, there is apprehension about making mistakes. This person prefers isolation, is deficient in organizational ability.

When spacing between lines is exceptionally narrow, thought-processes are apt to be muddled, and there's a lack of reserve in relationships with others. Organizational ability is "cluttered."

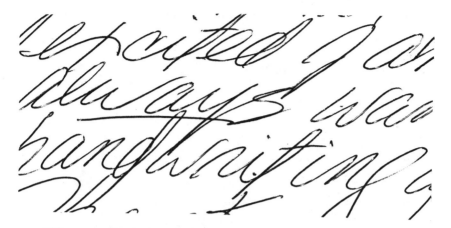

When spacing is crowded to the point of overlap, thought-processes are apt to be confused and disordered, relationship with others is impulsive and uninhibited, and organizational ability ranges from "unorganized" to "disorganized."

WORD-SPACING

The spacing between words is unconscious action, indicative of mental processes and sociability—or lack of it. Average spacing suggests objectivity and discretion in social relationships.

Exceptionally wide spacing between words usually signifies an "intellectual" person who avoids social contacts.

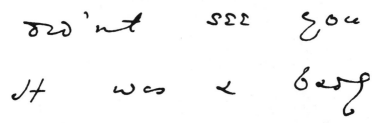

Extremely narrow word-spacing means self-confidence, with extrovert tendencies, and dependence on others.

Variable word-spacing—wide sometimes, narrow other times—points to instability in thinking and emotions.

Handwriting that shows horizontal expansion in both letter and forms, and in letter-spacing, generally reveals a forthright personality, free and uninhibited in social contacts. But if too wide, the writer is an intruder. If expansion is occasional, it indicates awkwardness, even if not prolonged.

If letters are too narrow, we look for a timid, suspicious inhibited individual.

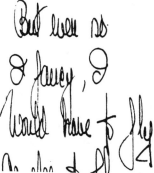

However, some handwriting showing expansion is merely an effect of wide spacing of narrow letters. This characteristic points to conflict. It may indicate freedom in social contacts, accompanied by inhibitions in the more intimate relationships. These inhibitions cause frustration and various kinds of illness because of a lack of understanding, closed-mindedness, lack of communication.

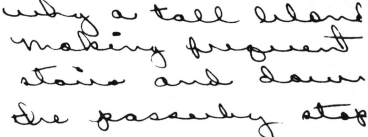

Imbalance in the use of space—inconsistent spacing, crowding in spots, looseness at other points—reveals conflict.

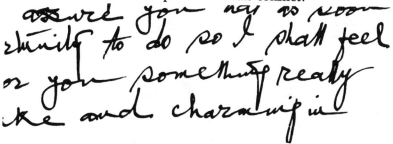

1. *Uniform line-spacing* has its roots in a sense of order. This is an attribute of the person possessing not only the ability to organize daily routine, but the capacity to assimilate emotional

experiences and maintain essential integrity.

2. The writing of a hypersensitive, moody person shows extreme variability in alignment. There is a kind of irregular alignment in which lines begin with ample word and letter-spacing, then end in a tangle of pinched, distorted characters piled almost on top of each other. It indicates the individual who dawdles in the morning and rushes about helter-skelter by evening, or who spends lavishly the first of the month, and lives like a miser at the end of the month. This type of person may consume the time and patience of others with preliminaries, and then at the moment of departure is obliged to blurt out what should have been said at the start.

Please send of my handwriting address below.

Please send me something large

Ample evidence has accumulated from medical studies that a cheerful individual resists disease more readily than does the "sour-puss." Spontaneous laughter is good therapy! A hearty laugh stimulates liver, lungs, heart, intestines, stomach, glands. Yawning and stretching helps relax the body, clears the mind, stimulates the brain, sharpens reflexes and eases excess tension.

Willie worked today

the body helps eapa

Charles Atlas

Closely crowded words indicate an absence of a feeling for privacy, insecurity, unsure ego, and a craving for contacts. Such a person doesn't "keep his distance" but is at one's heels much of the time. Narrow letters, combined with extreme compaction within words, reflect anxiety, sometimes obsession.

Since direction is further interpreted in terms of time, the movement of each letter embodies *past*, *present*, and *future*. We must observe the beginning and the end of each letter to determine whether the movement is a continuous advance toward the right. Letter and word are part of the sentence, and continuity of advance, or lack of it, gives clues as to whether the orientation is toward the past, the present, or the future.

In some handwriting an *ascendant* gradation in size appears — the terminal letter in each word is larger than the initial one. This often occurs in the writing of children and childlike adults. These people manifest a limited understanding of others.

As a rule, the writing of mature adults contains a *descendant* gradation. This points to diplomacy, insight, and capacity to function effectively in interpersonal relationships.

So far you agree

'e too large for worry, noble for anger, too strong · fear, and too happy to

MARGINS

Among the many factors in writing over which the writer has complete control is the left margin. The center of the page may be considered the present; the left of the page, the past; and the extreme right, the future. *If the left margin is extremely narrow,* it's a safe bet the writer is emotionally tied to the past. A narrow left margin symbolizes the irreversible—that what has happened in that person's life is irrevocable, the negative pattern cannot be changed. And the choice is made to cling to these concrete memories.

Consistent adherence to an *exceptionally narrow left margin* indicates a measure of withdrawal—for a variety of reasons. It may be because of fear of the present and the future—a condition of general repression. Because withdrawal is consistent and extreme, it cannot be considered accidental. Such a writer chooses and prefers to cling to the past. This tendency may be considered a form of repression.

The individual steeped in tradition is much more likely to maintain a *narrow left margin* because again this signifies a tie with the past. While existing in the present, the past *is* the present for such a personality.

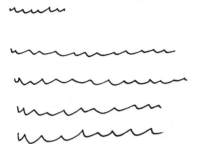

Conversely, a wide left margin bespeaks an individual who prefers to ignore the past, refuses to retreat into it, and is uninfluenced by it. One who has had an unpleasant past often leaves a wide margin, somehow symbolizing a barrier through which the past cannot penetrate or threaten.

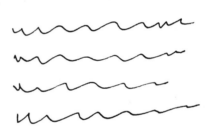

A left margin that becomes wider as writing progresses down the sheet indicates a person who, while closely attracted or attached to the past, is capable of overcoming the attraction in day-to-day involvement.

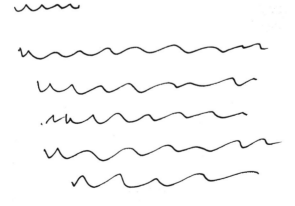

A well-regulated right margin, not limited by the vertical edge of the paper, is a sure indicator of the well-regulated, consistent individual. Most of this person's behavior can be foretold with accuracy. Such a person adheres to prescribed limits, down to the most minute detail. When very little space is left between the edge of the writing and the paper's edge, we are certain the writer is not afraid of the future, since the right side represents the future. There may be uncertainties, questions in the mind, but there's no fear about facing and penetrating the future. Could this trait also mean the person is generous? On the contrary, the space has been monopolized for self. We wouldn't call such an individual "stingy," but he may be classified as conservative, thrifty.

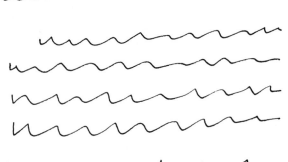

The opposite-type personality leaves a wide right margin, indicating hesitancy and uncertainty about the future.

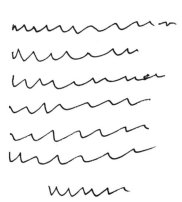

CREATIVITY

The creative person—able to visualize and create, construct with the hands—reveals this ability in broad, rounded, or flat-topped *m*'s, *n*'s, *r*'s. Persons possessing this personality trait are able to learn, and retain—*when they understand the reasoning or logic behind the rule.* Seldom do they learn by rote. They usually have artistic, musical, or literary talent. If you're one of these people, you do not form conclusions hastily, but instead methodically gather information on which to base a decision.

EXPLORATORY TRAIT

The explorer boldly ventures into the unknown, not dependent on others for opinions, preferring to obtain facts at the source. This trait is revealed in the inverted "v" structure pointing up from the base line.

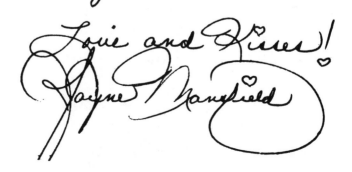

PERCEPTION

Needle-points reflect ability to grasp ideas. Comprehension comes seemingly without effort. The individual with this trait may become impatient with someone who takes too much time "getting to the point." The fast thinker with instant comprehension reveals this trait in needlelike points on *m, n, h, r, s*. The rate of speed at which one thinks is not the determining factor in intelligence, it should be added.

We are at a critical point: either we do what we must to win this election NOW or we allow our country to continue down the path that will lead to socialism.

Ronald Reagan

Franklin D. Roosevelt

can understand

THE ANALYTICAL TYPE

The analytical mind sifts ideas and facts, determining benefits and drawbacks. Possessing ability to reason, the analytical mind deals solely with the material at hand—evidenced in handwriting by the "v" structure pointing down toward base line.

and — Tommy Cinkovitch (& Dept.) is coming back from

what you have learned,

getting nothing but theory,

PRIDE

Pride—reasonable or justifiable self-respect—comes to us after we've accomplished something we believe is worthwhile. Roy Gardiner was proud of being "a good train-robber." Some people are proud of heritage, social or economic position. Whatever gives us cause to be proud (and it could be strong character rather than material possessions), it's evidenced in handwriting by high *d* and *t* stems--two to three times higher than lower-case letters—either looped, or retraced.

The degree of pride is revealed by the height of the stems in relation to the rest of the writing. Excessive to the point of conceit (more than three times higher than lower-case letters), it becomes a liability. Extending into the abstract, the elongated stems are suggestive of a mental quality, removed from daily experiences. The vain person first is proud of an accomplishment, then becomes conceited. This results from mental indulgence in the achievement long after its worth has been fully recognized, and perhaps appreciated by others. Vanity is to revel in "past glory." It's an unhealthy mental state, not conducive to action, and certainly may be classified as destructive. It could be the consequence of parental lack of recognition and appreciation of accomplishments during childhood.

HOW DO YOU CROSS YOUR T's?

WILLPOWER

A straight stroke betokens force and drive, while a curved stroke infers flexibility, a tendency to yield. The *t*-crossing indicates objective or purpose — ability to set goals and plan. If the stroke is unyielding, purpose is strong and definite. If we find a measure of yielding, we know the objective drive is somewhat diluted.

We pay special attention to *t*-bars because they're a significant guidepost — like a compass. Are we in control of our destiny or do we allow the winds of chance to determine it? *T*-bars are made long, short, consistently strong, weak, precise, controlled. They denote strength, weakness, enthusiasm, accelerated momentum, impatience, shallowness, dominance, sarcasm, procrastination, domineering tendency, temper. Here are specimens of what we're talking about.

Balance, precision, steadiness, orderliness:

Considerable loss of precision:

Drive delayed, becoming ineffective:

Impatience:

T-bar fades, lack of persistence:

Impatience, uncontrolled and unpredictable — a form of restlessness:

Enthusiasm, greater personal interest in projects; overdone, it becomes a detractive force, depleting vitality.

Lessened enthusiasm, but optimism added. This person leans more toward intangible thoughts and beliefs than pragmatism:

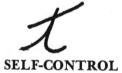

SELF-CONTROL

Presence of the curved stroke toward the base line on both ends tells us the writer is making an effort at self control:

The *t*-bar which moves toward the material, momentarily changes course, but terminates in a downward direction, indicates a stronger attraction to material values. It could mirror humor, artistic capabilities, and to a degree indicates a lack of ambition, coupled with an undertone of insecurity in the abstract. Thus, this person strives to return to the material realm.

The picture changes in this bar. Optimism plays an important role, as well as the feeling of security. This positive influence manifests in a sense of humor, and willingness to nurture artistic abilities.

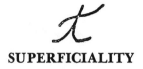

SUPERFICIALITY

The inverted curve in this stroke points to feelings of indifference, or superficiality. Each end is further into the abstract. Starting the stroke in the abstract, the writer makes an effort to approach the material; but as the movement progresses, it yields to the stronger abstract influence.

THE DOMINATING PERSONALITY

This bar compels others because of its strength, particularly if supported by positive qualities. Others clearly must bow before its greater conviction. Shown here is more strength and ability. A *domineering* bar (below) reflects *force and sharpness.* The dominating bar is not brutal unless supported by many negatives, including selfishness.

THE DOMINEERING PERSONALITY

Wanting our own way, and expecting it: Domineering. How do we accomplish it? By nagging, whining, tears, sarcasm, temper, demanding, cursing, threatening, even physical violence. *This trait is a defense mechanism.*

DIGNITY

Retraced *d*- and *t*-stems indicate dignity. The individual carries himself easily, perhaps gracefully; but at the same time there's a certain amount of restraint. Dignity implies quality, discretion, consideration of others. Dignity enables one to stand tall, to carry the head high, even in times of emotional stress. Mere possession of dignity, however, does not place one above reproach. There are dignified criminals.

$$\mathcal{d} \quad \mathcal{t}$$

INDEPENDENCE

When *d*- or *t*-stems are short by comparison, regardless of size of the overall writing, the trait of independence is present. Such a quality borders on stubbornness—it's difficult to distinguish between the two in personality behavior. Stubbornness is a state of mind. Independence, however, carries a more material connotation, suggestive of more activity than stubbornness. The independent individual is more likely to *do* as he pleases, than to *think* as he pleases.

state of mind

state of mind

The Esoteric
Constitution of Man

The mere looking at externals is a matter for clowns, but the intuition of internals is a secret which belongs to physicians. — Paracelsus

Since ancient times man has held the belief that his physical body is simply the externalization of more subtle vehicles of manifestation. References to these invisible bodies are to be found in a wide variety of texts originating in China, India, Egypt, and ancient Greece. The Bible too refers frequently to the subtle anatomy of man, particularly in *The Revelation of St. John.*

It is fashionable today to dismiss such ancient beliefs as mere superstition, holding them as impracticable and beyond any scientific proof. Curiously enough many of these writings, some of which are over five thousand years old, show clearly that the ancient seers and philosophers had a remarkably detailed knowledge of the anatomy and physiology of the human nervous and endocrine systems—two areas in which modern science still has much to learn.

For the most part, radionic practitioners accept that man has a subtle anatomy, but there are few who view it as they would the physical body, that is, as having definite form and clearly defined functions. It tends to become a rather vague amorphous mass into which healing rates are projected, and practitioners place a limit on their effectiveness by using this approach.

There is a passage in Wachsmuth's book, *The Etheric Formative Forces in Cosmos, Earth and Man*, which is relevant to this point. He writes:

"In future the art of healing will rest upon a knowledge of the etheric in Nature and in man.... If one views these realities not abstractly, but in the living man in their world relationship, one then arrives at new forms of knowledge in pathology and therapy in the art of healing."

This passage not only indicates the future trend of the healing arts when they emerge from the present materialism, but clearly shows that the reality of the etheric forces and the subtle workings of nature must not be viewed in a pseudo-mystical manner, but in a practical context relevant to the living man. The vague idea of the subtle bodies underlying the physical form must be replaced with the knowledge of structures which have a definite relationship to the visible anatomy and its physiological processes.

Man manifests as a triplicity of spirit, soul and body. The pure spirit is analagous to the Father in heaven, the soul is the high self, and the body the low self. The low self is likewise triple in nature, consisting of the mental body, the emotional or astral body, and the physical etheric body.

The theory of the etheric body stems primarily from the Eastern esoteric teachings, in which the emphasis is placed upon the subtle nature of man. The oriental asserts that the objective physical body is but the outward manifestation of inner subjective energies.

This etheric body, consisting of fine energy threads or lines of force and light, is the archetype upon which the dense physical form is built. It can best be described as a field of energy that underlies every cell and atom of the physical body, permeating and interpenetrating every part of it, and extending beyond to form a part of what is commonly called the health aura. The Bible speaks of it as the "Golden Bowl." To those with deeper vision it is often seen as a web or network animated with a golden light.

This etheric framework consists of material drawn from the four ethers, which is built into a specific form. The network of fine tubular threadlike channels, commonly known as the nadis, are related to the cerebro-spinal and sympathetic nervous systems. These channels, depending upon the quality of energy they carry, pass to certain areas of the body via the chakras, or centers of force within the etheric body.

The integral unit formed by the etheric and physical bodies is basically the most important vehicle of man, as it connects the physical world with the subtle worlds. Through it the five senses are able to function on the physical plane, and progressively it is able to register the impact of energies flowing to it from the higher realms.

There is in the human body a symbol of the distinction between the higher etheric and lower physical levels. It is quite simply the diaphragm, which separates the upper cavity of the body, containing the organs concerned with activities analogous to those of a spiritual nature, from the viscera which are concerned with the more mundane but necessary pursuits of a material nature.

The etheric body has three basic functions, all closely interrelated. It acts as a receiver of energies, an assimilator of energies and as a transmitter of energies. If each of these functions is maintained in a state of balance, then the physical body reflects this interchange of energies as a state of good health. The key to health lies in the correct reception, assimilation and distribution of energies.

Now let us consider the physical body. It must never be forgotten that this is but the earthly habitation of the soul, in which we dwell only for a short time in order that we may be able to contact the world for the purpose of gaining experience and knowledge. Without too much identifying ourselves with our bodies we should treat them with respect and care, so that they may be healthy and last the longer to do our work.

Thus we see that our conquest of disease will mainly depend on the following: Firstly, the realisation of the divinity within our nature and our consequent power to overcome all that is wrong; secondly, the knowledge that the basic cause of disease is due to disharmony between the personality and the soul; thirdly, our willingness and ability to discover the fault which is causing such a conflict; and fourthly, the removal of any such fault by developing the opposing virtue.

The duty of the healing art will be to assist us to the necessary knowledge and means by which we may overcome our maladies, and in addition to this to administer such remedies as will strengthen our mental and physical bodies and give us greater opportunities of victory. Then shall we indeed be capable of attacking disease at its very base with real hope of success. The medical school of the future will not particularly interest itself in the ultimate results and products of disease, nor will it pay so much attention to actual physical lesions, or administer drugs and chemicals merely for the sake of palliating our symptoms; but knowing the true cause of sickness, and aware that the obvious physical results are secondary, it will concentrate its efforts upon bringing about that harmony between body, mind and soul which results in the relief and cure of disease. And in such cases as are undertaken early enough the correction of the mind will avert the imminent illness.

Amongst the types of remedies that will be used will be those obtained from the most beautiful plants and herbs to be found in the pharmacy of nature, such as have been divinely enriched with healing powers for the mind and body of man.

For our own part we must practice peace, harmony, individuality and firmness of purpose, and we must increasingly develop the knowledge that in essence we are of divine origin, children of the Creator, and thus have within us, if we will but develop it, as in time we ultimately surely must, the power to attain perfection. And this reality must increase within us until it becomes the most outstanding feature of our existence. We must steadfastly practice peace, imagining our minds as a lake ever to be kept calm, without waves, or even ripples, to disturb its tranquility, and gradually develop this state of peace until no event of life, no circumstance, no other personality is able under any condition to ruffle the surface of that lake or raise within us any feelings of irritability, depression or doubt. It will materially help to set apart a short time each day to think quietly of the beauty of peace and the benefits of calmness, and to realise that it is neither by worrying nor hurrying that we accomplish most; but by calm, quiet thought and action we become more efficient in all we undertake. To harmonize our conduct in this life in accordance with the wishes of our own soul, and to remain in such a state of peace that the trials and disturbances of the world leave us unruffled, is a great attainment indeed and brings to us that peace which passeth understanding. Though at first it may seem to be beyond our dreams, it is in reality, with patience and perseverance, within the reach of us all.

Glands, Emotions, and Handwriting

Just as our sensory organs were placed by an all-wise Creator in the upper-portion of our bodies, so do emotions originate from that part of the organism.

We do not identify odors or flavors with our legs, nor do we see with them. The eyes do the seeing, through the brain, which instructs the legs on what movements to make. The brain is the instrument with which we think, see, hear, smell, taste, feel. These senses, in action, may motivate the action of the legs, the arms, or some other part of the body, but except for the sense of touch, neither our arms nor our legs recognize odors, colors, or sound.

When emotionally stirred, we may reach with our arms to grasp a loved one. Or if emotionally stirred in a negative way, our arms and legs may be used to ward off intrusion—to act aggressively against another. But the emotion that motivates such use of our legs and arms is not within the appendages, but in the upper part of the body—the brain.

Food is digested in the stomach, but aside from hunger pangs, it does not of itself "desire" food. Desire originates with one or more of the sensory organs. Food tastes "good" or "bad." If the odor attracts us, desire is aroused. An odor that is offensive (to our perception), may result in nausea. (Though what may "smell good" to one person, might be anathema to another. Some people, for example, don't like the odor of codfish, or Limburger cheese.) The stomach has its function, but it does not "desire" except as directed by the sense which creates the desire.

Likewise, the sex organs: Located below the waistline, their function is to procreate, and they do not go into action unless aroused by the mind, and/or the sensory organs.

Located within the skull at the top of the body, the key to all functions is the brain, responsible for translating the messages sent by the sensory organs — the nose, the eyes, the ears, the mouth — into smell, sight, sound, taste.

Repeating — since the emotions originate in the upper body, so do we experience the sensation of "love" in the upper part of the body, perhaps reaching out with the arms (upper body) to touch or embrace a dear one.

The "pulse of being" is represented by our nervous system (switchboard). The act of inhaling is a centripetal force; exhaling utilizes the principle of centrifugal force, or movement.

YOUR WRITING MIRRORS YOUR BODY

Every letter formation (unconsciously perhaps) becomes a record of inner drives that are difficult-to-impossible to reveal by other methods. Letter-formation likewise faithfully portrays body structure: Head, trunk, legs. The base line of handwriting may be likened to the waistline, at the navel.

Over-development of one zone invariably occurs at the expense of one or both the other zones. The consequence of such one-sided excesses is experienced in lack of inner balance — a condition culminating in "explosive" behavior.

MUNDANE AREA

About half the letters in the alphabet are formed in what the graphologist calls the "mundane" area (Webster defines it: "of, relating to, or characteristic of the world; having no concern for the ideal or heavenly.") The 13 letters in this category are *a*, *c*, *e*, *i*, *m*, *n*, *o*, *r*, *s*, *u*, *v*, *w*, *x*. These letter formations relate to our interest in the world we live in — interpersonal relationships, career, human affairs, current events — earthly concerns rather than celestial. The top of the letter structure in this area is referred to as the mental, or thinking, line, where the writing indicates mental acuity, and such intellectual interests as creating, exploring, investigating.

Gland	Area Governed
Pineal	Upper brain. Right eye.
Pituitary	Lower brain. Left eye. Ears. Nose. Nervous system.
Thyroid	Bronchial and vocal apparatus. Lungs. Alimentary canal.
Thymus	Heart. Blood. Vagus nerve. Circulatory system.
Pancreas	Stomach. Liver. Gall bladder. Nervous system.
Gonads	Reproductive system.
Adrenals	Spinal column. Kidneys.

MORAL, SPIRITUAL AREA

The moral, spiritual area is represented by the upper zone, where the letters *b*, *d*, *f*, *h*, *k*, *l*, *t* normally extend. This area may be regarded as having a relationship to the upper part of the torso and the head.

MATERIAL, PHYSICAL NEEDS

Letter structures below the base line (*f*, *g*, *p*, *q*, *y*, *z*) relate to the writer's material interests, including the expression of sexual needs. Below the waistline of the body lie the intestinal-digestive system, bladder, and gonads (sex organs). Besides their reproductive function, the gonads secrete hormones necessary for correct metabolism and muscular strength. We can characterize the gonads as organs representing the creative energy of the body. At its purely physical level—sex, appetite, physical desires—this energy can be constructively employed. Misused, it can be destructive.

The doors of the subconscious (control center, solar plexus) are opened to this energy, enabling the subconscious mind to rise to the pineal gland in the brain—believed by some to be "the seat of the Great Mind—the Christ-consciousness." This energy then is transmitted to other centers of the body via the pituitary, or "master gland," which, under direction of the hypothalamus, regulates such body processes as growth, reproduction, and various metabolic activities.

ADRENAL GLANDS (Protection)

The adrenal glands—one covering the upper surface of each kidney—produce life-essential hormones. For handwriting-analysis purposes, the adrenals are located in the mundane area of the small-letter fomations, as well as the upper-zone letters. It is in the mundane area that most of the positive-negative emotions, fears, and repressions of emotions, are identified. At times of extreme stress—perhaps fighting or fleeing from an agressor, or when performing a strenuous physical act in emergency—these glands secrete adrenalin, providing the necessary additional energy to cope with the crisis.

Under control of the sympathetic nervous system, and functioning in conjunction with it, the adrenal medulla is intimately related to adjustments of the body in response to emotional states. Intense emotional reactions trigger the release of the hormones norepinephrine and epinephrine. Reserve power is wedded to emotional climate, which can be controlled and directed by conscious thought. This energy, when guided by positive thought, generates goodwill, joy, courage, patience, unselfishness, and the ability to be quiet and calm by listening to and heeding the "inner voice." Contrariwise, negative thoughts direct this force to generate such emotions as anger, hate, fear, prejudice, selfishness.

Positive emotions increase energy; negative emotions lower the energy level. And to compound the ill effects, negative emotional responses activate the glandular system to manufacture more toxins. (These emotions are evident in handwriting.) Emotional temperament—serene, disciplined, or "stormy"—is the basis of character traits. Emotions affect glands by increasing or decreasing blood and energy circulation. Constant negative use of energy brings about emotional instability, high blood pressure, certain types of heart disease. The chronic worrier, having burned up the energy supply, winds up in a permanent state of exhaustion. Negative emotions prevent the body from renewing and rebuilding itself. To harbor animosities or resentments is to lock in the toxins, preventing the body from renewing and rebuilding itself. The antidote—which you've guessed by this time: Cultivation of spiritual thoughts which give birth to goal orientation, courage, persistence, patience, and the art of being able to listen, to others as well as self.

CULTIVATE LAUGHTER

Anatomy Of a Laugh
In their rush to see why humor is good for you, scientists uncover the wild gymnastics of joy. —Robert Brody

Laughing Goes Institutional

At DeKalb General Hospital in Decatur, Georgia, patients head to "The Lively Room" in search of serious mirth.

In several Missouri jails, offenders try to straighten out through a rehabilitation program that helps shed light on their problems with cartoon humor.

At the Ethel Percy Andrus Gerontology Center in Los Angeles, volunteers have developed a handbook on how to use funny materials—cartoons, limericks, books, records, and movies—in caring for the elderly.

With the offical word now out that humor is healthy for you, laughing is going institutional: In hospitals, nursing homes, hospices and prisons. The basic idea is to create an atmosphere conducive to healing. Through this holistic approach, patients (and prisoners) can form an upbeat attitude that just might ward off illness (and criminal impulses).

At the Veterans Administration Hospital in Sepulveda, California, for instance, comedian Bill Dana performs for patients as author Norman Cousins plays stright man. "Bill gets them going until the room is filled with one continuous roar," Cousins says.

Most patients report leaving the 45-minute laugh fests relieved of the pain they otherwise suffer.

"Laughter interrupts the 'panic cycle' of an illness," Cousins explains. "In blocking panic, it prevents constriction of blood vessels and negative biochemical changes."

"Humor—and the entire range of positive emotions, such as faith and hope—can play an important role in medical treatment," Cousins says. "But it's wrong to encourage sick people to regard laughter as a cure-all or an easy substitute for competent medical treatment."

Laughter is partly chemical. When you laugh, you stimulate your endocrine system, including the pituitary gland. Laughing itself prompts you to secrete hormones that rouse you to high-frequency alertness. These hormones, called catecholamines, include epinephrine, norepinephrine, and dopamine. As they circulate in your blood, they drive the laugh by stimulating your heart, other glands and hormones, and your breathing, and by contracting and relaxing your arteries. The pituitary gland may also stimulate release of endorphins and encephalins, natural painkillers that are chemical cousins to opiates, such as morphine and heroin. As you laugh, the right hemisphere of your brain—that which governs emotion and spurs creativity—is more chemically active than usual. During laughter, the two hemispheres seem to get on unusually well.

Infants start laughing around the tenth week after birth. At that stage, they laugh reflexively, at surprises or in relief at such bodily sensations as passing gas or voiding the bowels. By the 16th week or so, they're already laughing about once an hour.

Since the central nervous system is still under development in the newborn, infants have little appreciation of humor. Soon enough, they get the hang of laughing at discomforts that previously brought on crying. Kids develop a tolerance of—and capacity to convert into laughter—all manner of tension (depending on their parents). At age four, they're laughing about every four minutes, mostly at the slapstick humor popular in playing.

Now you're on the verge of laughing, ready to vent your sense of fun. The zygomatic muscles with which your face makes expressions are going into contortions. You seem almost to grimace. On command from the cortex, your abdominal, lumbar, internal intercostal, subcostal and transverse thoracic muscles contract like fists. Your vocal cord muscles, designed for intelligible sound, cannot coordinate. Your glottis and larynx open, relaxed and ready to vibrate. Your diaphragm tenses in anticipation of respiratory spasms. Air in your body billows till you feel pressure building in your lungs. [Trying to hold in a laugh is no less than a violation against nature—rarely successful.]

Abruptly, your breathing is interrupted for a station break. Your lower jaw vibrates. A blast of air gusts into your trachea, flinging mucus against the walls of your windpipe. Pandemonium! Out comes your laugh, in some cases clocked at 70 miles an hour. You issue a strange machine-gun sound, almost a violent bark.

A robust laugh gives your diaphragm, thorax, abdomen, heart, lungs and maybe even the liver, a brief workout, Doctor Viola Fry finds. Laughing with gusto turns your body into a big vibrator and performs an internal massage. Your muscles tighten, relax and thereby grow stronger. Thanks to a pulmonary-cardiac reflex, your pulse can double from, say, 60 to 120. Your systolic blood pressure can shoot from a norm of 120 to 200 during laugh tumult. Laughing is aerobic. Norman Cousins calls it "inner jogging." (Laughercise, anyone?)

Laughter as a formula for health is an old idea. Henri de Mondeville, a 13th-century surgeon, told jokes to patients emerging from operations. In the 16th century, English educator Richard Mulcaster advised laughter was the right medicine for head colds and melancholy, especially if you tickled under the armpits. Here in America, the Ojibway Indians had doctor-clowns, called *windigokan*, who performed antics to heal the sick.

THYMUS GLAND (Metabolism)

The handwriting analyst views the thyroid as a gland representing will power and psychic sensitivity. The presence (or lack) of this quality is recognized principally by the length, weight, and position of the *t*-bar. Psychic, intuitive, or "sixth sense" ability is evidenced in writing by open-flowing breaks between letters or words. The *t*-bar is the clue to the writer's strength of character, endurance, and will power. Selfish use of the will is said to result in hyperthyroidism—production of excess thyroxin causing nervousness and excitability. Non-use of the will, on the other hand, results in hypothyroidism—apathy saps vitality.

HEAL THYSELF

An explanation of the real course and care of disease,
by Edward Bock, M.B., B.S., D.P.H.

Disease will never be cured or eradicated by present materialistic methods, for the simple reason that disease in its origin is not material.

The state of boredom is responsible for the admittance into ourselves of much more disease than would be generally realised, and as it tends today to occur early in life, so the maladies associated with it tend to appear at a younger age. Such a condition cannot occur if we acknowledge the truth of our divinity, our mission in the world, and thereby possess the joy of gaining experience and helping others. The antidote for boredom is to take an active and lively interest in all around us, to study life throughout the whole day, to learn and learn and learn from our fellows and from the occurrences in life the truth that lies behind all things, to lose ourselves in the art of gaining knowledge and experience, and to watch for opportunities we may use to the advantage of a fellow-traveller. Thus every moment of our work and play will bring with it a zeal for learning, a desire to experience real things, real adventures and deeds worthwhile, and as we develop this faculty we shall find that we are regaining the power of obtaining joy from the smallest incidents—that occurrences we have previously regarded as commonplace or of dull monotony will become the opportunity for research and adventure. It is in the simple things of life—the simple things because they are nearer the great truth—that real pleasure is to be found.

Another fundamental help to us is to put away all fear. Fear in reality holds no place in the natural human kingdom, since the divinity within us, which is ourself, is unconquerable and immortal, and if we could but realise it we, as children of God, have nothing of which to be afraid. In materialistic ages fear naturally increases in earthly possessions (whether they be of the body itself or external riches), for if such things be our world, since they are so transient, so difficult to obtain, and so impossible to hold save for a brief spell, they arouse in us the utmost anxiety lest we miss an opportunity of grasping them while we may—and we must of necessity live in a constant state of fear, conscious or subconscious, because in our inner self we know that such possessions may at any moment be snatched from us and that at the most we can only hold them for a brief life.

In this age the fear of disease has developed until it has become a great power for harm, because it opens the door to those things we dread and makes it easier for their admission. Such fear is really self-interest. When we are earnestly absorbed in the welfare of others there is no time to be apprehensive of personal maladies. Fear at the present time is playing a great part in intensifying disease, and modern science has increased the reign of terror by spreading abroad to the general public its discoveries, which as yet are but half-truths. The knowledge of bacteria and the various germs associated with disease has played havoc in the minds of tens of thousands of people, and by the dread aroused in them has in itself rendered them more susceptible to attack. While lower forms of life, such as bacteria, may play a part in or be associated with physical disease, they constitute by no means the whole truth of the problem, as can be demonstrated scientifically or by everyday occurrences. There is a factor which science is unable to explain on physical grounds, and that is why some people become affected by disease whilst others escape, although both classes may be open to the same possibility of infection. Materialism forgets that there is a factor above the physical plane which in the ordinary course of life protects or renders susceptible any particular individual with regard to disease, of whatever nature it may be. Fear, by its depressing effect on our mentality, thus causing disharmony in our physical and magnetic bodies, paves the way for invasion, and if bacteria and such physical means were the sure and only cause of disease, then indeed there might be but little encouragement not to be afraid. But when we realise that in the worst epidemics only a proportion of those exposed to infection are attacked and that, as we have already seen, the real cause of disease lies in our own personality and is within our control, then have we reason to go about without dread and fearless, knowing that the remedy lies within ourselves. We can put all fear of physical means alone as a cause of disease out of our minds, knowing that such anxiety merely renders us susceptible, and that if we are endeavoring to bring harmony into our personality we need anticipate illness no more than we dread being struck by lightning or hit by a fragment of a falling meteor.

The chakras have three main functions.

****

First — To vitalize the physical body.

Second — To bring about the development of self consciousness.

Third — To transmit spiritual energy in order to bring the individual into a state of spiritual being.

****

The chakras in the etheric body are to be found in various states of activity.

The following diagram illustrates the position of the seven major chakras, their glandular correspondences and the areas of the physical body directly governed by them. It should always be remembered that each chakra, although only present in subtle matter, externalizes itself on the physical plane as an endocrine gland, just as the nadis materialize as the nervous system. There are some texts which stress very strongly that the physical nerve plexii and endocrine glands should not be confused with the chakras. It is true that they should not be confused with the centers; on the other hand it is not correct to divorce the endocrine system from the chakras, as the latter are simply an extension of the former. It cannot be too strongly stated that the subtle anatomy directly relates to the physical. Acting as though they were separate factors only leads to a distorted view of the total man.

The Seven Major Spinal Chakras

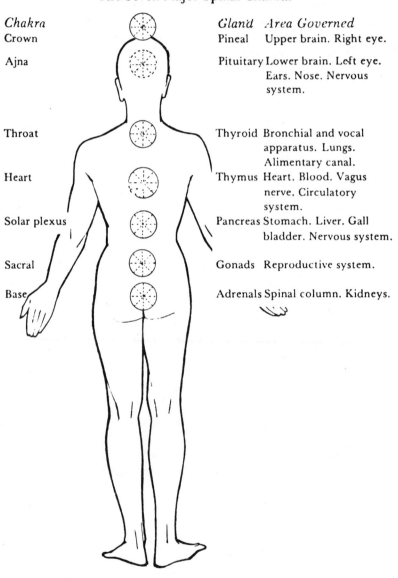

Chakra	Gland	Area Governed
Crown	Pineal	Upper brain. Right eye.
Ajna	Pituitary	Lower brain. Left eye. Ears. Nose. Nervous system.
Throat	Thyroid	Bronchial and vocal apparatus. Lungs. Alimentary canal.
Heart	Thymus	Heart. Blood. Vagus nerve. Circulatory system.
Solar plexus	Pancreas	Stomach. Liver. Gall bladder. Nervous system.
Sacral	Gonads	Reproductive system.
Base	Adrenals	Spinal column. Kidneys.

SELF-CONTROL

If you're one of those "composed" individuals who always seem to be in charge of your emotions, able to restrain impulses through use of will power, the handwriting analyst will spot the trait in the way you cross your *t*'s: with an arched *t*-bar.

be interested

The Inter-

ri Society

Other clues to self-control are a pattern of evenness in base line, spacing, fairly even margins, and nonconflict between loops in upper and lower zones.

thoughts. A man thinks -
tinctively - and then he ac
rights - all that he thinks
does - have their start in
feels and when you kno.

CONSISTENCY

The person consistent in thoughts and actions reveals the trait in handwriting that maintains evenness in the middle zone; correct base line slant; consistent letter- and word-spacing. Firm, even pressure translates into firm responses. Light pressure is a signal that the person shows minimal interest in what's going on around her or him.

ANXIETY

Anxiety states are observed in handwriting as contracted in the center zone, with cramped, narrow letter formations. Frequently (but not always), the writing slants backward. Narrowness, compressed letters, backward slant, overemphasis on upper and lower loops, varying pressures, firm and weak *t*-bars, combine to give the writing the appearance of disharmony. And it points to an individual suffering from a variety of conflicting tendencies and considerable internalized anxiety.

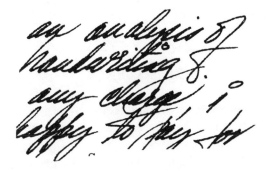

ULTRA-CONSERVATISM (Fear of Change)

Not to be confused with penuriousness, selfishness, or fear of expression, ultraconservatism is a product of rigid thought and behavior. The poor soul afflicted with this emotional distortion fears new situations with a paranoic fervor, oblivious to the reality that *change is a natural condition of man's environment, and adjustment to change is vital and essential*, not only to growth and development, but to survival. This stultifying fear of and resistance to change affects all areas of personality, warps mental habits, and inhibits achievement. It is expressed in handwritng by compressed spaces between letter structures, and retracing of some formations.

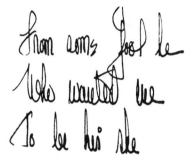

SENSE OF HUMOR

Nearly everybody enjoys the person with a sense of humor—able to see the funny side of a sorry mess, to laugh at oneself—fun to be around such a person, right? If you're gifted with that faculty, you're fortunate—it's one of the best shields against tension buildup. The trait can be identified by the initial flourish that blends into the following stroke, with no angle between strokes, thus:

BALANCE AND MODERATION

The romance and challenge of life—getting the most out of it—is achieved by avoiding extremes. There's nothing wrong with the desire for eating, drinking, mating. But everything is wrong with gluttony, alcoholism, promiscuity. Premature aging is the price we pay for indulgence in *emotional storms*.

to thine own self be true

Graphotherapy Exercises

So you've taken on some attitude habits that turned into emotional syndromes and at times make life something less than pleasant?

And you'd like to get rid of these mental barnacles?

Praise the Lord! You *can* weed them out of your personality garden! It'll take time, patience, and bulldog determination — but *you don't have to live with destructive thought-emotion processes*, not for a cotton-picking minute!

The formula is simple: Translate desire into action. These pages list some of the common mischief-makers you can go to work on — today! One suggestion: Take them one at a time. Select the trait you most want to change, and go to work on it with pencil or ballpoint.

Figure out how many minutes you can spare, what time of day best suits your schedule. then *do it* come hell or high water! No excuses or alibis for missing it a single day! Get the exercise or exercises in even if you have to wait till bedtime, if it's been that kind of a day. Think of it as a session with your doctor (only, if you're faithful, you'll eventually find less need for his services), or as a music lesson (unless that turns you off). Make it serious, and keep it fun. Don't begrudge the time — in fact, say a little thank-you prayer for being led to take on this therapy assignment! If you're not grateful at the start, you will be when the light shows at the end of the tunnel!

There may be times in the beginning when you think it doesn't make sense. But just as sure as you get up in the morning, if you'll treat the project as soberly as you expect to be treated by your doctor, you'll win a victory. And who, more than yourself, would be a more challenging adversary? And a more elated victor?

Interwoven into every human experience are emotions. A baby's cry arouses an emotional response — positive or negative; a rooster's crowing stimulates emotions; the sight of a fruit-laden tree or flower-laden bush evokes emotional response (delight, perhaps, or guilt because they need watering or pruning); a spouse's smile — or frown — stirs emotions; the sound of the sea booming against rocks, a gull's cry, a desert rock, a waitress' warmth or indifference — all communication, whether verbal, visual or touch, elicits emotional response, pleasant or not-so-pleasant, soothing or irritating. The list is endless.

We identify emotions by the feelings they kindle in us: joy, sorrow, love, hate, expectancy, disillusionment, disgust, fear, to name a few.

High on the list of destructive emotions is fear. In fact, it probably rates at the top of the devil list, since there are so many gradations and manifestations of this emotion.

Fear results from real or imagined threats to our security — physical, mental, spiritual, material. Unless we consciously and deliberately throw the rascal out, refuse to acknowledge its presence, it will take over — dominate behavior, stifle creative activity, and stymie development of an integrated personality. It is a demon in every sense of the word!

One of the reactions to fear impulses is repression and suppression of emotions. Natural or normal expression is stymied when we subconsciously or consciously exclude from memory unwanted thoughts, feelings and experiences. Repression is an escape mechanism serving as an emotional balance-wheel. While we seemingly achieve a measure of "security" by repressing emotions, we also effectively block creativity and the germination of new ideas (imagination). To exercise this control deliberately and consciously is suppression. Repression is a constant process, suppression occurs periodically. Crowded handwriting is a symbol of the control of expression.

We recognize it in handwriting thus:

REPRESSION: *M*'s, *n*'s consistently retraced (subconsciously):

repression is a constant
process and is found
mostly in the retracing
of the m and n

much money
components

SUPPRESSION: *M*'s, *n*'s occasionally retraced, not consistently:

suppression indicated
m's + n's are occasionally
retraced :
Release from these
negative impulses
is important

Release from these negative impulses is a first step in "opening" ourselves to the freedom of balanced psyche: centeredness. If you happen to be among those needing and wanting release, this exercise will turn the trick. Discipline yourself to weave it into your daily "musts" and expect results!

EXERCISE: _____

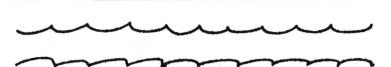

There may be a little of this trait in most of us—some think it adds zest to life—but the desire for variety and frequent change of scenery suggests a distaste for, perhaps even a fear of, some element or condition of our environment. We're not talking about the yen occasionally to "get away from it all," but rather the compulsion to constantly want to be on the go, unable to really enjoy the homefires. If you're thus afflicted, it will show up in the lower extensions of g, j, y, z.

The extremely long stroke that does not return to base line is evidence that one is running away from reality—there seems to be no anchor.

Narrow, compressed loops signal an absence of imagination, consequently very few friends.

And here is a sample of handwriting telling us that since the below-base-line loop is less than half the height of the letter in the middle zone, the writer finds security in routine, is easily satisfied, spends most of the time "in a rut."

loop less than half the height of the letter in the middle zone

Readjusting our mental state to face reality and remove the fear that inhibits imaginative, creative endeavor can be accomplished by putting our mind and attention to the following exercise. Remember—it took time to form the trait you now want to eradicate, and you can't expect instant results. But results you'll get if you stay with it.

a b c d e f g h i j k l m n o p q r s t u v w x y z egegegegegegeg

CLANNISHNESS

Clannishness is identified in handwriting by a tight, restricted loop at the bottom of *g, j, y, z*. Indicating a feeling of insecurity, it's frequently the result of an unhappy social environment. If you happen to be saddled with this personality quirk, you are fiercely loyal to friends, but possessive, unwilling to share them. The degree of clannishness is measured by the size of the loop. An abnormally small loop indicates close friends are limited to one or two. The larger the loop, the wider the circle of friends. However, if the return stroke is not brought back to base line, the elitist, possessive trait known as clannishness still is present.

g j y z g j y z

Assuming you'd like to move away from insecurity feelings, manifested among other ways in possessiveness toward a chosen few, if you'd like to experience the exhilaration of variety that comes through a wide circle of friends and acquaintances, set aside a few minutes each day and do this exercise. Don't cheat yourself by skipping a "lesson"—make a game of it. You're due for some surprises!

g g g j j j y y y
z z z

JEALOUSY

Jealousy—fear of not being needed, wanted, or loved—is a distressing personality condition, not only for the person suffering from the trait, but to the others involved. Carried to the extreme, it is expressed in violence, sometimes deadly.

Without question, the human being's most vital need is to experience love. Peanuts says it's our "security blanket." To be loved gives us confidence, purpose, self-esteem—the entire package of "good feelings." A person torn with jealousy might very well be loved by the one against whom the jealous feelings are being projected, but this doesn't come through; jealousy blinds us to reality. The jealous individual is emotionally unstable and, when we get right down to the nitty-gritty, *does not really love* the friend or mate of whom she or he is jealous. If love is mature and genuine, there's no room for jealousy. It's as simple as that.

In handwriting, the "jealousy loop" starts with a "back-to-self" stroke, telling us the writer is wrapped up in self, and features self. The jealous person wants to be important to one person only—a mark of frustration, since it is normal to include many individuals in one's circle of associates. The jealous person is insecure, *feels* unable to cope with a situation that actually should pose no problem.

m   *n*   *h*   *b*   *d*

Weeding out this "baddie" *is* possible. You don't have to live with the satanic insecurity feelings expressed in ravaging jealousy—feelings that do you more harm psychologically, spiritually, and eventually physically, than other ways you may punish yourself. Resolve that you *want* to free yourself of this demon, then take action. The following exercise, performed regularly and with total concentration, is the key to freedom from jealousy.

m   *n*   *h*   *b*   *d*

VANITY

Vanity, inflated self-esteem, stems from feelings of rejection and injured pride. It serves as compensation for the real—or fancied—disapproval of associates. Webster describes vanity as the "relative or absolute lack of values." The vain person overestimates ability, makes promises with no intention of fulfillment. In handwriting, vanity is exemplified by *d*- and *t*-stems more than three times the height of the writer's *m*'s and *n*'s.

meant done

You may not think that a bit of vanity is all that bad—but perhaps if you could see yourself as others see you when you're flaunting that emotional response to injured pride, you might just say, "Enough! I'll stamp it out!" If that's your choice here's how:

the the the did did

STINGINESS

The close-fisted, penurious person actually suffers from fear of want. The instinct of self-preservation is one of the most powerful forces in the human experience. Freedom from want produces (at least it *should* produce) security. Fear of want breeds insecurity feelings. One of the blessings of the feeling of genuine security is generosity: The need to share oneself and one's possessions. Stinginess is a by-product of acute fear of material deprivation. Hence the inability to share oneself and possessions. This trait reveals itself in excessively crowded handwriting—no generous spacing between letters, no generous endings.

Generosity is indicated by wide spacing between letters and words, long endings in the broad circle letters, and open *e*'s.

words, if I sent ample of another writing, would you — to send me your

Perhaps you *like* the feeling of seeming security that comes from stubbornly hanging on to all your earthly goods? And you couldn't care less whether others see you as "stingy"? In our beautiful world of free choice, that position is fine, but the only thing is, you don't do your spiritual, emotional, or physical states any favor by nursing fear feelings of want and insecurity. It's been proved repeatedly that this emotion produces harmful effects. If you'd like to trade it off for the healthy feeling of security, this is the way to do it. Guaranteed results.

eeeeeeeeeeeee eeeeeeeeee

DAYDREAMING

Wishful-thinking reverie—daydreaming—is an escape mechanism. Inhibited by fears, the person thus afflicted cannot experience self-realization, and so often resorts to escape in the fantasy world, where he is unchallenged. Likewise, no problems are solved. Perhaps the only virtue of this personality quirk is that daydreaming may seem to make the burden bearable. Daydreaming shows up in handwriting in a weak and/or "floating" *t*-bar:

that floating t bar

Here's another trait you may think you enjoy: Fantasizing, escaping from the problems of the real world. But if you'd like to connect with reality—and you can take my word, it's a pretty satisfying experience—this exercise will help you do it:

the the the the

SUPERFICIALITY

We may not see ourselves thus, but if one of the facets of our personality is shallowness—lacking in depth of knowledge, reasoning, emotions, character—we actually are trying to escape from problems, unwilling to face reality. The shallow approach to life suggests a lack of purpose, lack of achievement drive. Behind this trait is our old friend, *fear*. Responsibilities are frightening, and if circumstances become "really rough," the person so afflicted will not hesitate to withdraw rather than face the problem. By no means does this characteristic imply impaired mentality. It does mean, however, that under intense pressure, one might take the drastic measure of deserting responsibilities and family.

The trait is evidenced in inverted or dish-shaped *t*-bars.

t

The beautiful thing about graphotherapy is: You're "the doctor." *You* initiate the changes and work on them mentally, just as you must do if you use the services of the professional psychologist or psychiatrist. The exercise below is aimed at rooting out another aspect of *fear* which may be showing up in your life as the trait known as shallowness, or superficiality. If you're convinced this would be better out of your life, apply yourself to the following bit of retraining—and it won't hurt to say, sing, or shout, "Praise God!"

tttttttt

DECEPTIVENESS

The person who considers it advantageous to employ deceit in dealings with others—whether actually to cheat, or rationalized as a "tactical resource"—may be said to be also deceiving himself.

Deceptiveness in character is revealed in handwriting when loops are made in the "circle letters"—*a, o, g, d*—the letters said to represent thoughts and ideas.

Open loop: the writer is frank, talks easily.

can do no harm

Initial loop: Reveals self-deception.

she were always unaware of her problem

Double loop: can be positive or negative. Individual will deceive or mislead others, but entire handwriting must be analyzed to determine whether it's positive or negative.

lauging is good for one

Loop tied at right side: Indicates secrecy—writer will withhold information. May be positive or negative, depending on other traits. Note: This loop is "positive," with high form level—ethical, honest, intelligent, generous, ambitious, determined. The professional person (doctor, diplomat, etc.) may use deceit and secrecy to protect. Individuals who are oversensitive or overly considerate may overdo this trait as a means of self-protection. A balance between secrecy and talkativeness is desirable, particularly in an executive secretary or persons working with the public.

The professional person person may use

Double hook formation within circle: This represents evasion. The writer evades truth to retain or acquire what he desires—objects, services, information, ideas.

The double hook reveals evasion

Whether you want to change this trait is your decision. I can assure you that if you do have a habit of telling white lies—or if you engage in more serious evasions of truth—you'll *feel* better toward yourself, and others, by "telling it like it is." Deceitfulness does not go undetected, though one may go for years, perhaps forever, without being challenged. The trait demands cover-up. Cover-up is stress-producing. And by now you know what stress can do to health. So, if you'd like to trade that habit for one of straightforwardness, tackle this exercise, stick with it, and you'll become a new person in this particular personality area.

a a a o o o d d d

g g g a o d g

ARGUMENTATIVENESS

The person who doesn't get through a day without at least an argument or two really is suffering from a compulsion to defend ideas and actions—a defense mechanism against criticism. In handwriting, the stroke related to this trait is in the lower-case *p*, the lower loop denoting physical action. Made with an initial stroke that penetrates or explores the abstract area, the writer is combining thought with action.

A lower-case *p* considered "normal" is written thus:

play

Resentment of presumedly being imposed upon supports the argumentative attitude:

please please

The imaginative person (upper loop) defends ideas more vigorously:

pull

If you'd like to change a defensive attitude and become a better-integrated person, this exercise, practiced conscientiously and regularly, will do the job:

p p p p

IRRITABILITY

Irritability—nervousness—is another defensive trait usually triggered by tensions. If this shows in your handwriting, there could be many reasons: restlessness, job dissatisfaction, delays, impatience with yourself and others. A result of friction—

disharmony—it stems from excessive nervous tension. In handwriting, irritability is revealed by distorted *i* and *j* dots:

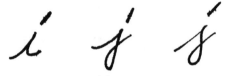

When the jabs are directed toward the writer it signifies irritation with self:

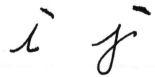

If directed forward, it tells the analyst the irritation inflicted is on others. A forward, downward jab reveals a domineering, nagging personality.

Irritability—defensiveness—is another albatross we can do without. It's an energy-waster, and unchecked can lead to health problems. If you agree, and want to oust this trait, the how-to follows:

TEMPER

Most of us possess a "temper"—described by Webster as "a mood dominated by a single strong emotion such as anger"—a character trait that can get us into trouble if not controlled.

Temper is a method of resistance, and of dubious value in coping with a problem. If anything, it magnifies the problem. A tragic example was a tavern fight reported in Los Angeles: One man died and his attacker was imprisoned, over a glass of spilled beer! The news report said the glass was accidentally knocked from the table by a 20-year-old patron who apologized and replaced it, but that wasn't enough for the other young man. He started arguing, there was a scuffle, the emotionally-disturbed beer drinker produced a knife and inflicted a fatal gash. An extreme example, perhaps, but not at all an isolated case of violent behavior when emotions run wild.

If you "have a temper," you're probably on the lookout for an act or expression you think is directed against you. The aroused temper facilitates striking out in self-protection. It means, too, that you are "weak" in defense against perceived imposition by others, and the temper is a release of indignation and hostility. You also may show temper if deterred from doing what you *will* to do, your frustration resulting in anger and fear, and loss of control of will power.

Temper is revealed in handwriting if the *t*-bar follows the stem rather than crossing it:

Another clue to temper is the beginning "tick" stroke:

If you'd like to bring that temper under control—or teach others how—here's the exercise that will do it, if faithfully performed:

INDEPENDENCE

The independent thinker is a nonconformist who insists on setting standards without much caring what others may think. In handwriting this trait is identified through a short *d*-stem, indicating independence in conduct of personal affairs, including dress and behavior:

indicating independence

A short *t*-stem indicates independence in choice of career goals:

short t stem indicates independence in career and goals

A measure of independence can be an asset — a leadership trait. Carried to extremes, and exerted on weak-willed companions, it could produce an outlaw, of course.

independence — asset or outlaw? Look to companions that that did did

AGGRESSIVENESS

This trait shows up in handwriting by a marked increase in pressure on forward-moving final strokes, particularly the lower-loop structures. When hostility traits are present, aggressiveness is a character liability.

are you going by

This exercise is designed to retrain the subconscious to direct achievement drive toward less abrasive behavior:

by going

DEFIANCE

The defiant individual is quick to resist forces that may infringe on freedom of action. Defensive, of course, it may be the consequence of environment in which authority has been misused: Home, school, job. Usually it is directed against authority figures. The trait may not surface in an open display of rebellion.

Defiance is revealed in formation of lower-case *k*, the last section inflated disproportionately:

take work

When part of the "buckle" is in the mundane area, part in the abstract area, reality is involved, and the trait is likely to be expressed by belligerence or rebellion:

work buck

Defiance also shows up in formation of the printed *k*:

work buckle

Here's how this trait is brought under control by those who want to:

work take buckle

RESENTMENT

Hostility traits are not escape nor adjustment mechanisms. They are counterattacks to resist the forces that stand between the individual and his desire to exercise free will, choose goals, and attempt to achieve them. Resentment resists intrusion into the right to think and act freely. If this trait is detected in your writing, it means your "guard is up"—you suspect your rights are being threatened and you're on the alert for possible impositions.

If you happen to be burdened with resentment, unfortunately it will influence other traits. For example, instead of "forgiving and forgetting," past injustices linger in the memory bank, coloring today's thoughts and acts. The person possessing this trait is a potential troublemaker in a group. And it isn't only the others who suffer. One misses exciting opportunities simply because of the feeling (usually misplaced) that the other fellow intends to take advantage. Uncurbed, resentment can become an overwhelming negative force within one's personality. It brings no solutions, only new problems. In essence, this characteristic is the unwillingness, or inability, to forgive. Resentment is identified in handwriting by the inflexible strokes attached to the circle letters starting at or below the base line: *a, c, d, o, g, m, w, y.*

Aggressiveness also is indicated by inflexible strokes at or below base line and attached to the *h, k, t*—"springboard" strokes:

You'll reap a rich reward if you vow to rid your personality of resentment. You may think you get pleasure nursing old should-be-forgotten grievances, real or imaginary, but if you'll uproot them and cast them out, you'll find new vistas opening, new pleasures coming into your life, a new feeling of freedom and peace of mind that can't be bought with all the money in the world. Practice this exercise diligently, and gather in the harvest!

a a c d d g g
m m n n o w w
h h k r t d

SARCASM

Sarcasm is an outlet for hostility. It reveals frustration, and feelings of inadequacy. If this trait shows in your writing (and I hope it doesn't), it points to a sharp, biting spirit that gets satisfaction from verbally punishing another person. Existence of the trait reveals a basically ineffective person in some specific area or areas. Its indiscriminate use *does not* win friends and influence people.

In handwriting, a sarcastic bent is disclosed by a sharp-pointed *t*-bar:

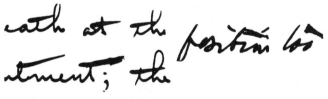

We see here that the stroke started out firmly and ended weakly, as if to say, "you don't follow through." This builds frustration, which then is expressed through sarcasm directed at others. The degree varies — it may be mild, or it may be so strong it becomes malicious behavior, particularly if resentment is combined with sensuality (revealed in heavy, clogged script).

If you'd like to eliminate indecisiveness, you can do it by faithfully performing this exercise:

a b c d e f g h i
j k l m n o p q r
s t u v w x y z

PERSISTENCE

We don't want to sound moralistic, but one of the gifts we can cultivate—to realize almost unlimited benefits over the long haul—is plain old persistence! If you're fortunate enough to possess this trait, you fall into the group who "never say die," who bounce right back after a temporary defeat.

Depending on other factors in the writing, this trait can be a positive or negative force. It is a positive force in the well-organized person when combined with moral and ethical attitudes, a good mind, and generosity.

Persistence is revealed in an upstroke that moves to the left, forming a loop as it returns in a downward swing and crosses itself and the downstroke from which it originated, as in:

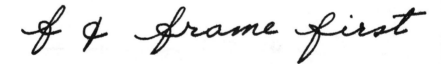

While it might sound old-fashioned to preach its value, I unhesitatingly recommend cultivation of persistence to anyone—goal-oriented or not. The feelings of frustration, the nagging guilt-feelings occasioned by the knowledge "we have left undone those things which we ought to have done," (to quote *The Book of Common Prayer*), are not conducive to long-term health, psychologically or physically. The following exercise will help you cultivate the quality of persistence:

Persistence in a positive sense is part of the personality of a person who is well-organized, intelligent, cultured, possesses pride in achievement, and maintains harmonious relationships.

This trait when negatively displayed symbolizes repression, low self-esteem, a low level of self-motivation, and limited spiritual concepts.

TENACITY

A near-relative of persistence, surely, is tenacity—the habit of stubbornly clinging to ideas, plans, or possessions, hanging on to what we have. It can be a real negative, and is not a habit to cultivate. In handwriting it's indicated by a hook at the end of a letter formation, at the end of strokes within words.

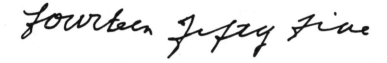

PROCRASTINATION

If your personality repertoire contains the trait of procrastination—putting off till tomorrow what could and should be done today—it tells the analyst you are likely to be harboring such negative traits as hypersensitivity, self-consciousness, self-underestimation, indecisiveness. If you fear criticism, or lack confidence in your ability to perform, procrastination becomes the mechanism to delay decisions, action. It is an ego defense to evade the possibility of failure and ridicule. And, of course, it generates frustration because the inevitable is merely delayed.

This trait is identified by a *t*-bar at the left of the stem, falling short of reaching or crossing it:

procrastinate

And if you tend to delay decisions or attention to details, it shows up in the dotting of the *i* at the left of the stem:

it is interesting

You'll feel better psychologically—and eventually even physically—if you decide to relegate this habit to the garbage can. It can be done by conscientious performance of this exercise:

relegate this habit to

SELF-CONSCIOUSNESS

Self-consciousness—fear of ridicule—may have its roots in early childhood experiences during the awkward period: skinny or fat perhaps, "buck" teeth maybe, or freckles—whatever was a little *different* from the norm, causing playmates, friends, and/or family to tease and ridicule. While those who point the finger of ridicule don't realize it, these gestures make a deep impression on the sensitive child. The fear of being ridiculed registers in the subconscious, affecting behavior into adolescence and adulthood.

Our fears are related to insecurities that threaten the homeostasis of our ego. We have a deep, abiding need to be accepted for *our* standards, *our* way of life. If, through earlier conditioning, we feel inadequate, if we get the idea that somehow we don't measure up socially, we become a victim of self-consciousness. And we fear humiliation and ridicule. We feel much more comfortable in familiar surroundings and among acquaintances who accept us regardless of "peculiarities." We're aware of feeling self-conscious in unfamiliar situations.

How do we recognize this character trait in handwriting? When the final hump of *m* and *n* extends above the others. The higher the hump, the more pronounced the trait.

We feel inadequate when somehow we could measure up.

How can we overcome self-consciousness? By retraining the subconscious through this simple exercise:

we can overcome self-consciousness

TIMIDITY

Self-consciousness and fear of expressing oneself are components of another trait: Timidity. Another of the social fears, it blocks full development of personality. It is destructive in that one's potential is not realized—a tragic consequence when you analyze it! If you are among those afflicted with this trait, you're destined to remain immature in certain areas. You are inclined to mentally withdraw, keep your feelings and desires to yourself to cloak feelings of inferiority, lack of confidence. This is a curse, really, because inhibitions are personality cripplers, robbing one of the satisfactions and joys of fulfillment.

As noted earlier, self-consciousness is betrayed in the formation of the final hump of *m* and *n*—higher than the predecessors. Lack of confidence is signaled by low *t*-bars on the stem. Fear of expressing oneself is detected in retraced *m*'s and *n*'s, as well as circle letters (tied to a compulsion for secrecy).

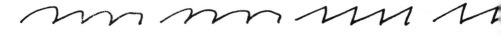

Release from the shackles of timidity is achieved—if you desire a fuller life—by applying yourself to this exercise:

SUBMISSIVE NATURE

The yielding, submissive nature more often is a detriment than a blessing. Since the world is not yet dominated by love as the strongest force utilized by humans, the person who lets others "get away with it," becomes the proverbial doormat. Intellect has nothing to do with it, either. You can be brilliant, yet submissive to the point of severely damaging your personality and your desires for fulfillment. So you take the path of least resistance and go along with the suggestions of others, regardless of how they may conflict with your standards and creative urges. About the only time this trait can be said to serve a useful purpose is when possessed to some degree by an executive who tends to be inflexible on most issues. The trait in such a personality "softens" her or him on occasion, creating a more acceptable employer-employee relationship.

The yielding nature is revealed in rounded (known as "soft") strokes. Such letters lack definite formation.

I am writing this for
analysis research proje
indications in writi

If you recognize this quality in your own personality, and would like to achieve more balance and become capable of running your own show—saying "no" when the inner voice directs—incorporate this exercise into your daily routine for as long as necessary to make the switch from "yes-man" to your own man (or woman!).

capitals this is

SUPER-SENSITIVITY

Fear of disapproval—super-sensitivity—develops from the feeling of threatened security (usually imagined). It can have a basis in fact, however: The children of too many parents hear criticism constantly, rarely praise. This is another assault on the psyche that can be more damaging than a spanking, and far-reaching in personality distortion. Whatever the cause, we must deal with the consequence now—behavior characterized by constant suspicion that someone is or will hurt us. We all know such persons, poor souls. They're not easy to be around

The person who builds up mental images of the reasons others have to cause hurt or harm can be identified via handwriting by enclosures in the loops and circle letters. When a loop appears in the upper extension of lower-case *d* and *t*—where it does not belong—the writer is imagining reasons others disapprove of his or her way of life.

experience both contacting
all levels of distributi
broad background whi wr

Retraced *d*'s and *t*'s suggest a sense of dignity, but not sensitivity to criticism.

First I would like coming and speaking u class. I appreciated th

Sensitiveness can be so exaggerated by imagination (loops) that the writer has completely forgotten the reason for the hurt:

can be ordered from the and all details of each crime

If you happen to be overly sensitive, and want to escape from the trap, here's the recipe:

dont loops ts and ds

SELF-UNDERESTIMATION

Fear of failure—self-underestimation, a sense of inferiority—oftentimes is acquired early in life, the consequence of parental failure to show the approval and acceptance so vital to a new life. Self-esteem is a basic element in the secure, well-adjusted personality, and it doesn't develop when a child is subjected to a barrage of indiscreet, indiscriminate criticism and punishment by parents and teachers. Fear of failure is another destructive emotional block that cripples initiative and creative impulses and stymies development of one's potential (and each of us does have potential, don't ever forget it!). Fear of failure means fear of not achieving a goal. Saddled with this fear, one simply doesn't *try*. It hurts to fail, so it's more comfortable not to make the effort—a devastating trait, responsible for the withering of creativity, beautiful potential, fulfilling life.

So how do we identify this fear? By *t*-bars low on the stem:

the tall thin man went to the theatre

And how do we dump this trait once and for all? By concentrating on this easy exercise—worth more than gold, believe me.

its rattle tattle and bottle

DEPRESSION

Have you ever known a person who built up resentment against a co-worker, employer, relative, or friend because of a feeling that she or he had been treated "unfairly"? This syndrome can lead straight to depression; the more often the "tape" is played, the more intense the depressed state. Some people hang on to every bad experience, every insult (real or presumed), any possible injury as prized possessions. There is also the type who, like a "blame blotter," accepts responsibility for everything that goes wrong. The only beneficiary of this practice of replaying the "tapes" of hurts and injustices inflicted by others is the pharmaceutical industry which cashes in on sales of tranquilizers and antidepressants.

The person who persists in nursing resentments springing from "unfair" treatment winds up with physical disorder—dis-ease—showing up. When you permit yourself to brood over hurt feelings, there's a reaction in the intestines—a kink develops. Prolonged brooding, without making an effort to "clear the air" through rational communication, results eventually in a permanent intestinal disorder—the kinks become fixed. And if the mood becomes bitter, unforgiving, you're a good bet for liver trouble or gallstones. Goiter and other throat problems can be a consequence of feelings of inadequacy and submissive helplessness, all wrapped up in the package labeled "negativism."

I once watched a woman make herself seriously ill because of her resentment over being placed on a four-day week due to temporary financial stress. In her mind the issue was further aggravated when her assistant was laid off. This resentment (and she actually acknowledged this as the source of the ensuing trouble) built up to a point at which the doctor ordered her to rest. Had he been a skilled psychologist or psychiatrist, she might have been brought out of it by simply facing the whole thing and talking it out. She is a fastidious worker, a competent secretary, and "her own worst enemy." She was wanted and needed at her desk—which she knew—but damned if she would give them the satisfaction of her services after the "unfair" treatment! So her illness progressed and her relations with her family disintegrated. She was a prospect for the ultimate withdrawal—death—until she was fortunate enough to find a doctor who helped her get her mental house in order. And another dear friend, unable to shake the *belief* that someone whom she loved no longer cared, did, in fact, allow herself to withdraw from the real world until, sadly, she did die!

How to get out of this trap? How to reverse the downward trend from "slow burn" to deep depression, to physical disability? Along with massive doses of "stop-feeling-sorry-for-yourself" (the world's full of beautiful people *when we turn ourselves around*), start finding things in your life to be thankful for. Look at God's creation with new eyes and ears. It's magnificent! So are the creatures within it—from the multilegged insects and feathered two-leggers to Homo sapiens!

And try this exercise in corrective graphotherapy. You *can* turn yourself around, you *can* start loving living—a precious inheritance we so often overlook as we sink into the abyss of despondency and self-pity. Learn to forgive and forget.

At M. F. U. we did not have a policy of showing the horses to any great extent. I hauled to 4 shows, 3 of which were futurities. Out of 11 classes entered we placed in the top 5 in all but two classes.

MENTAL ILLNESS

In the early stages, mental illness may be detected by increasing illegibility, increasing irregularities. There may be omission of letters or syllables, varied slants, lines swinging in various directions.

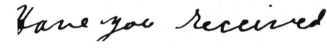

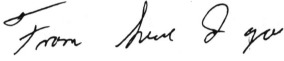

If this is uncovered in someone's writing — or in your own — take immediate steps to reverse the trend. The following exercise, practiced diligently, will start you on the road back to a more normally balanced, fruitful, fulfilling life:

need control and a fairly even baseline

NARROW-MINDEDNESS

If this trait—unfortunately not uncommon—is revealed in handwriting, and if there's a desire to move away from a provincial, hypercritical, perhaps bigoted mind-frame, it can be accomplished through graphotherapy. (See exercise below.) The attitude or trait is indicated in writing by these narrowly formed letters: *e* (particularly in the lower-case *e*), *a*, *o*, *g*, *d*.

you kindly send
u, magazine. Jean
der, then what m ah

And narrowly formed upper and lower loops on these letters:

Pacific which won
to travel with wago
Mexico; and to the C.

EXERCISE: _____

eeee aaaa oooo dddd
lll hhh ggg yyy jjj

EMOTIONAL DISTURBANCE

The professional handwriting analyst detects an emotionally disturbed person through several different types of signals: Varying slants of letters; variations in pen or pencil pressure; inconsistency in *t*-bars; lines that waver and vacillate; lower loops may be too small, too large, or nonexistent; letters may be cramped or too widely spaced.

Severe anxiety is reflected by cramped or narrow middle-zone letters, or backward slant with narrow, compressed letter formations.

Release from this condition is possible by employing graphotherapy as indicated for individual emotional problems enumerated in this chapter—perhaps starting with the exercise to eliminate depression, repression, suppression, resentment, jealousy.

Suggestion: Take one trait at a time. Do the exercise 30 times each night for 30 minutes, or if convenient, do it morning and night. *Make it regular.* When it becomes part of the subconscious, you have conquered the problem. Make a game of it, and eventually—if you persist—you won't recognize the old you. Family, friends, will be talking about that "new woman," or "new man."

How To Improve Your Health by Changing Your Handwriting

Often you've heard someone say, "If a person has health, he has everything!"

With health, we can survive some pretty desperate situations. With health, we can rebuild a lost fortune; renew, repair, or create new human relationships important to us. With health, we can greet each new day with assurance, zest, the zingy feeling that makes you want to say, "It's great to be alive!"

As noted earlier in this book, there *is* a way to reach that goal—if you'd like life to be more stimulating, more fun. It's not a complicated procedure. The only requirements are *a desire to change*, and a measure of self-discipline.

Others have improved their health by changing their handwriting, and you can too. Here are the six simple rules guaranteed to bring about fundamental changes in your personality, your mental, your emotional, *and* your physical well being. Even if you work on only one, you'll experience improvement in your health.

Medical doctors tell us that most of our upset stomachs and headaches are a direct result of disturbed emotions: Fears, frustrations, guilt feelings, tensions. Try the following exercises.

Start with these warm-ups:

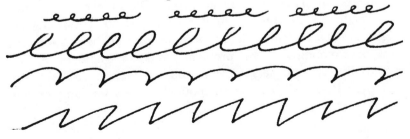

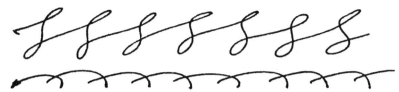

These six exercises, practiced regularly, will (1) improve your rhythm; (2) help release inner tension; (3) aid you in creating greater harmony and continuity in your everyday life.

THE SIX BASICS

Now you're ready for these six basic exercises. Work with them, follow them faithfully, and you will be amazed at what they'll do for you in terms of your health, and your ability to enjoy yourself and those around you:

1. *Open the 11 letters which should be open:*

2. *Close the two letters which should be closed:*

3. *Dot your i's:*

4. *Cross your t's:*

5. *Maintain even spacing of lines, not too far apart, not too close together:*

Too far apart:

Too close:

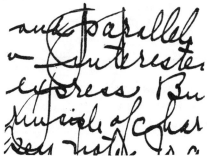

Good spacing:

Thank you for sending my
pendulum so promptly— I
am very well pleased with
it.

6. *Maintain consistent height and width of letters:*
Consistent height:

I am starting a small mail-
order herbal gift business. I
need small gold boxes, such

Inconsistent height:

another mental mechanism of a
is when a person is ~~is is~~
is he will be assassinated or

Consistent width:

you will have to make allow
ances. also, I have used the

Inconsistent width:

Which time I moved the "Jam to Clovis, Ca-near Fresno. I am so

A FEW CASE HISTORIES

John sought my opinion as to how he could get out of his rut. Employed as a designer for a large manufacturing company, he could see no chance for advancement.

His writing indicated that he was highly creative, artistic, and an original thinker. He had an exceptional personality, and was liked by fellow employees as well as by his supervisor.

I found that either he did not cross his *t*-bars, or the bars were weakly placed in every conceivable position. This was a clear signal that he did not set goals, did not plan his work or his future. He was just "floating." He was aware of this attitude, but did not know how to correct it. John also complained of headaches and hypertension. He was nervous, restless, and dissatisfied.

I gave him some exercises with a number of small t's, told him to think up other exercises with small t's, asked him to get a soft lead pencil and to cross those *t*-bars about two-thirds of the way up the stem, making the bar heavier than his regular writing. He was to do an exercise at least 30 times each day for 30 consecutive days. If he missed a day, he was to start over.

Two months later, this man gave notice of resignation at work. He had found a new job as chief engineer in another company. He stayed on that job about two years, then decided to form a nationwide consulting firm. He is a different person today, happy with his life, with his increased income, and with his extra leisure time. And he doesn't have those headaches or hypertension any more.

Joan is a successful secretary and a valuable employee for a small manufacturing firm. Extremely versatile, she fills in on many jobs in the office. For several years, however, she had been plagued with a problem of headaches and sick stomach, causing her inconvenience and time lost from her job.

She asked to have her handwriting analyzed. It indicated she

was warm-hearted, and interested in helping others to the point
that they frequently took advantage of her. She has a younger
sister who has a jealousy problem. Joan's writing revealed that she
bottled up her feelings, and was unable to talk to her sister about
problems as they developed. Her *m*'s and *n*'s were retraced

indicating inability to let her feelings come to the surface. She
also "tied up" the circle letters, indicating secrecy, or

not being frank and open about how she felt. She had had no
problem of tactlessness or being thoughtless of others.

Now she learned to open the circle letters and was astonished to
discover more harmony in her relationships, not only with her
sister, but with others. The headaches and sick stomachs are now a
thing of the past, and she and her sister are communicating,
talking about their problems. This has meant improvement for the
sister as well as for Joan.

Helen was tense and unhappy about her personal relationships
with friends and relatives when she came to me for a handwriting
analysis. Thirty-eight years old, she had been divorced six years,
and had a married daughter. Holding down a good job, Helen's
income was adequate, but she was bored with her job which
presented no challenges. After examining her handwriting I
concluded that the underlying reason for her discontent was her
excessive weight. She believed that friends and acquaintances were
avoiding her and did not like her. She was frustrated and jealous.

As in so many thousands of cases, her writing indicated
withdrawal—a retreat into her private shell: retracing the *h*'s, *k*'s,
m's, and *n*'s.

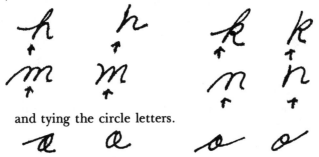

and tying the circle letters.

I asked her to open up *h*, *m*, and *n*, as well as *a*, *o*, *d*, and *g*. I also told her to get into the habit of greeting people with a smile and an outstretched hand, not to wait for them to make the first move. Now, she says, it's hard for her to believe "there are so many friendly people!" She's been promoted to a job with considerably more challenge. More contented, she snacked less, and easily lost the excess weight that was making her unhappy.

A supervisor for a small company, Miriam is a beautiful, kind, and loving person. She has a smile for everyone, and is well liked. As the weeks, months, and years passed, she became increasingly concerned with the pressures and deadlines of her job, and there were times when she actually wound up in the hospital with apparent symptoms of a heart attack.

She wanted me to analyze her handwriting. It revealed not only the lovely person she is, but also that she is exceptionally conscientious. However, as the deadlines rolled around she became more and more tense until something had to give—and actual illness resulted.

To release the tensions, I asked her to practice opening up *m*, *n*, *h*, and *k*. She found this difficult because the tensions were so entrenched. But she worked at it diligently, and as she succeeded, she became aware of a welcome difference in her health, and she's now better able to take things in stride.

Here's a sample of the change in the four letters, which came after much concentration:

old

m   n   h   k

new

m   n   h   k

Jane hated her mother-in-law with an intensity that was destroying her. She openly resented the attachment her husband felt for his mother. Jane's son was caught in the cross fire until he was a nervous wreck, vowing to leave home as soon as possible. Jane found every opportunity to speak with relatives and friends about her "horrible, vicious" mother-in-law. The more bitterly she complained, the more her husband defended his mother, and this merely added to her overwhelming resentment and feelings of martyrdom. As her emotions went out of control, her health deteriorated. Common were backaches, headaches, constipation, kidney trouble, high blood pressure, heart trouble.

She came to me for an analysis of her handwriting, and this proved to be a turning-point in her life. With counseling, and by working on the exercises in graphotherapy, she started gaining control of herself, and began to improve emotionally and physically. Here are some of the traits she had to change:

Lack of planning and sense of direction—wanting her husband to live her life for her, unwilling to stand on her own feet—indicated in weak, scattered *t*-bars:

Lack of decisiveness and ability to make decisions—indicated by weak endings of words:

Inability to communicate effectively, and bottling up emotions--indicated by retracing *m*, *n*, *h*, and *k*:

Lack of communication, and secretiveness—indicated by the tied circle letters:

She worked on these weaknesses with writing exercises, using the following letters:

Strong *t*-bars:

Decisive endings to words:

Open *m, n, h, k, o, a:*

A highly creative person, Jane could do anything with her hands. Now, with greater understanding, she is able to let go and let God. She is happier with her own accomplishments, and able to see the needs of others, including her mother-in-law. These changes, of course, have brought different responses from others. Her handwriting now shows much improvement, and her health has improved correspondingly.

Bob, 27, had worked his way up in his company from stock boy to supervisor of the shipping department. He complained of being blocked, with "nowhere to go" in his job, and he was having real problems getting along with his boss. Not overly popular with girls (according to him), he was convinced his personal life and career were unsuccessful. He was having more and more tension headaches, and severe eczema attacks.

He asked for an anlysis of his handwriting. It showed him strong in setting goals, but at the same time exceedingly domineering. This was indicated in the way he slanted *t*-bars downward, with a sharp point at the end:

It also showed him to be extremely critical of anything and everything he observed around him. Rarely, if ever, would he say anything good about another's performance. This trait was indicated by the *y* formations at the bottom of letters resting on the base line, and between letters on the base line:

His domineering behavior and critical observations turned people against him, and this in turn caused him resentment which was building up steadily, and was a major factor in the attacks of eczema. Resentment strokes are indicated by inflexible beginning strokes on circle letters in the middle zone:

Thoroughly unhappy with his condition, Bob resolved to try to correct his behavior. He applied himself diligently to these graphotherapy exercises:

He replaced domineering *t*-bars with these:

He endeavored to eliminate some of the analytical strokes in connecting letters:

He eliminated resentment strokes by writing his beginning strokes thus:

His health problems seemed to clear up almost overnight. He is making progress in social relationships and is noticeably happier.

It was because of my own experiences that I became a disciple of the science of graphotherapy.

I was fortunate to be part of a close-knit family. When we moved to California, I enrolled in a new school and had to make new friends. I was a shy person and this was the beginning of a series of emotionally-induced physical disturbances. But it was not until I took up graphology that I was able to master my whole being and enjoy almost perfect health. I have learned how to *not react* to disagreeable situations, and thus remain free of tension. With my interest in and practice of graphotherapy, it followed that I couldn't help but become more aware of myself as a spiritual being. This knowledge has its reward in good health and an insatiable enthusiasm for living.

When I got into graphology in 1959, I learned that I needed to concentrate on four areas. They were:

T-bars: mine were weak—meaning I was floating—not setting goals:

Looped *d* and *t*: I was too sensitive to criticism:

Retraced *m* and *n*, signifying that I was shy, uptight, causing constipation and eczema, and inhibiting me from expressing myself:

Tied *o* and *a*, meaning I was secretive, didn't express my feelings, which contributed also to inner tensions:

Through these exercises I was able to make the corrections in attitudes and behavior which truly transformed me into a liberated woman. Patterns of negativism were eliminated, and the energy-flow was redirected along positive pathways, through the following exercises:

T-bars were strengthened, and consistently placed on the *t*-stem:

Sensitivity to criticism was eradicated by forming *d* and *t* without loops:

Opened up *m* and *n*:

Opened up, for the most part, *a* and *o*:

After correcting the weakness shown in my writing, I was able to meet people and situations on a new basis. I learned to *not react*, while maintaining a lively interest in doing a good job, and I was freed from tension and the problems practically solved themselves. Truly!

I discovered that permitting myself to get upset blocked energy in my body and cut off a certain amount of contact with the source of all power. I learned that contact with power is contact with the source of ideas, and that energy then follows naturally and seemingly effortlessly. I learned to banish "energy leaks" by getting rid of negative thinking.

There is a natural rhythm to life. The person possessing assorted fears and inhibitions does not have a steady rhythm. I found that persons whose rhythm was interrupted by their own reactions were hard on machines, whether a typewriter, calculator, automobile, or whatever. Their machines were in the repair shop more frequently than were those operated by individuals with good rhythm. This lack of rhythm affects health adversely, particularly circulation. It can also be the source of accidents.

Results of my application of graphotherapy to my own condition have been most rewarding in that my rhythm is undisturbed, my energy unlimited, and every day is a new opportunity to enjoy a life of serenity, happiness, and health.

Appendices

Professional Organizations

American Association of Handwriting Analysts
1115 West Cossitt Avenue
La Grange, Illinois 60525

American Handwriting Analysis Foundation
Box 6201
San Jose, California 95150

Association of Professional Graphometrists
760 Market Street, Suite 315
San Francisco, California 94102

Berufsverband Geprufter Graphologen/Psychologen e.V.
Sitz Munchen, Cimbernstrasse 70c
8000 Munchen, West Germany

Canadian Graphology Association
101-1580 Haro Street
Vancouver, British Columbia V6G 1G6
Canada

Council of Graphological Societies
635 North Merrill
Park Ridge, Illinois 60068

Eastern Association for Handwriting Research
300 Sunset Terrace
Elmira, New York 14903

Federation Nationale des Graphologues Professionnels
2 bis rue Roger Simon Barboux
94110 Arcueil, France

Graphology League of Wisconsin
3621 South Clement Avenue
Milwaukee, Wisconsin 53207

The Graphology Society
Bell House Study Centre
Swanton Novers, Melton Constable
Norfolk NR24 2NW, England

Handwriting Analysts International
1504 West 29th Street
Davenport, Iowa 52804

Society for Integral Graphology
535 Perry Street
Sandusky, Ohio 44870

Schools and Colleges

Academy for Professional Graphometry
760 Market Street, Suite 315
San Francisco, California 94102

Felician College
206 South Main Street
Lodi, New Jersey 07644

Handwriting Analysis Workshop Unlimited
1166 El Solyo Avenue
Campbell, California 95008

Handwriting Consultants of San Diego
2410 Meadowlark Drive
San Diego, California 92123

Humanalysis Institute
1280 West Highway 96
St. Paul, Minnesota 55112

Institut National de Recherches Graphologiques
Le Pave du Roy
77780 Bourron Marlotte, France

Institut National de Caracterologie, Inc.
1888 rang St. Joseph
Chicoutimi, Quebec G7H 5A7,
Canada

Mercer County Community College
Mercer, Pennsylvania 16137

New School for Social Research
66 West 12th Street
New York, New York 10010

Trenton State University
Hillwood Lakes
Trenton, New Jersey 08625

San Jose State University
Washington Square
San Jose, California 95192

San Francisco State University
1600 Holloway Avenue
San Francisco, California 94132

Bibliography

Aab, Anna. *A Glimpse At Handwriting Analysis*. Lakemont, GA: C.S.A. Press, 1971.

    Teaching Yourself Handwriting Analysis. Lakemont, GA: C.S.A. Press, 1971.

Allport, Gordon W. *Pattern And Growth In Personality*. New York: Holt, Rinehart & Winston, 1961.

    et al. *Studies In Expressive Movement*. New York: Hafner Press, 1967.

Amend, Karen, and Mary Ruiz. *Handwriting Analysis: A Complete Basic Book*. North Hollywood, CA: Newcastle Publishing Co., 1980.

Arnheim, Rudolf. *Art And Visual Perception: A Psychology Of The Creative Eye*. Berkeley, CA: University of California Press, 1974.

    Visual Thinking. Berkeley, CA: University of California Press, 1969.

Bach, George R., and Herb Goldberg. *Creative Aggression: The Art Of Assertive Living.* New York: Avon Books, 1975.

Bauml, Franz H. *Die Handschrift.* Berlin: Walter de Gruyter & Co., Mouton Publishers, 1969.

Bloodworth, Venice. *Golden Keys To A Lifetime Of Living, 3rd edition.* Marina del Rey, CA: DeVorss & Co., 1968.

   Key To Yourself. Marina del Rey, CA: DeVorss & Co., 1980.

Bunker, M.N. *Handwriting Analysis: The Science Of Determining Personality By Graphoanalysis.* Chicago, IL: Nelson-Hall Publishers, 1966.

   What Handwriting Tells You: About Yourself, Your Friends, & Famous People. Chicago, IL: Nelson-Hall Publishers, 1966.

Byrd, Anita. *Handwriting Analysis.* New York: Arco Publishing, Inc., 1981.

Cammer, Leonard. *Up From Depression.* New York: Pocket Books, 1969.

Casewit, Curtis. *Graphology Handbook.* Rockport, MA: Para Research Inc., 1980.

Cerminara, Gina. *Many Mansions.* New York: William Morrow & Co., Inc., 1950.

Cole, Charlie. *Handwriting Analysis Workshop Unlimited.* Campbell, CA: E.C.F. Cole, 1961-68.

Cottrell, Marian. *Introduction To Handwriting Psychology.* Park Ridge, IL: Marian Cottrell, 1984.

   Understanding Adolescents Through Their Handwriting. Park Ridge, IL: Marian Cottrell, 1984.

Currer-Briggs, Noel, et al. *Handwriting Analysis In Business.* New York: Halsted Press, 1980.

de Sainte Colombe, Paul. *Grapho-Therapeutics: Pen And Pencil Therapy.* Hollywood, CA: Laurida Books Publishing Co., 1967.

Downey, June E. *Graphology & The Psychology Of Handwriting.* Baltimore: Warwick and York, Inc., 1919.

   The Will-Temperament & Its Testing. Philadelphia: Richard West, 1978.

Engel, Joel. *Handwriting Analysis Self-Taught.* New York: Elsevier-Nelson, 1981.

Erikson, Erik H. *Dimensions Of A New Identity.* New York: W.W. Norton & Co., Inc., 1979.

   Identity: Youth And Crisis. New York: W.W. Norton & Co., Inc., 1968.

Fallon, Hal. *How To Analyze Handwriting*. New York: Simon & Schuster, Inc., 1971.

Fink, David Harold. *Release From Nervous Tension*. New York: Pocket Books, 1962.

Flesch, Rudolf. *Why Johnny Can't Read & What You Can Do About It*. New York: Harper & Row, Publishers, Inc., 1966.
Why Johnny Still Can't Read: A New Look At The Scandal Of Our Schools. New York: Harper & Row, Publishers, Inc., 1981.

Fleming, Elizabeth. *Believe The Heart: Our Dyslexic Days*. San Francisco: Strawberry Hill Press, 1984.

French, William L. *Your Handwriting & What It Means*. San Bernardino, CA: The Borgo Press, 1980.

Friedenhain, Paula. *Write And Reveal: Interpretation Of Handwriting*. Atlantic Highlands, NJ: Humanities Press, Inc., 1973.

Frith, Henry. *Graphology: The Science Of Handwriting*. Blauvelt, NY: Steinerbooks, 1980.

Gardner, Ruth. *Graphology Student's Workbook, 2nd edition*. St. Paul, MN: Llewellyn Publications, 1975.

Gologie, Ralph V. *A Study In Symbolism: An Empirical Foundation Of Graphology*. Hixon, TN: Unique Books, 1973.

Grayson, David. *Better Understanding Your Child Through Handwriting*. LaGrange, IL: G B C Publishing, 1981.

Green, James, and David Lewis. *The Hidden Language Of Your Handwriting: The Remarkable New Science Of Graphology & What It Reveals About Personality & Health & Emotions*. New York: A & W Publishers, 1983.

Green, Jane Nugent. *You And Your Private I, 2nd edition*. St. Paul, MN: Jane Green, 1983.

Guthrie, Robert V. *Psychology In The World Today*. Reading, MA: Addison-Wesley Publishing Co., Inc., 1971.

Hagan, W. E. *Treatise On Disputed Handwriting & The Determination Of Genuine From Forged Signatures*. New York: A M S Press, Inc., 1981.

Hamilton, Beryl. *Measurement, Meaning, Message: The Cole Psychogram Method*. Campbell, CA: E.C.F. Cole, 1984.

Harris, Thomas A. *I'm O.K. — You're O.K.: A Practical Guide To Transactional Analysis*. New York: Harper & Row, Publishers, Inc., 1969.

Hartford, Huntington. *You Are What You Write*. New York: Macmillan Publishing Company, 1973.

Hearns, Rudolph S. *Handwriting: An Analysis Through Its Symbolism*. LaGrange, IL: American Association of Handwriting Analysts, 1973.

Neurotic Disorders And Depression As Revealed In Handwriting. Santee, CA: Graphology Consultants, 1984.

Self-Portraits In Autographs. New York: Carlton Press, 1981.

Hill, Barbara. *Graphology*. New York: St. Martin's Press, Inc., 1981.

Holder, Robert. *You Can Analyze Your Own Handwriting*. New York: The New American Library, Inc., 1982.

Holt, Arthur G. *Handwriting In Psychological Interpretations*. Springfield, IL: Charles C. Thomas, Publisher, 1974.

Hughes, Albert E. *What Your Handwriting Reveals*. North Hollywood, CA: Wilshire Book Company, 1978.

Ilg, Francis, et al. *Child Behavior, revised edition*. New York: Harper & Row, Publishers, Inc., 1981.

Jansen, Abraham. *Validation Of Graphological Judgements: An Experimental Study*. Hawthorne, NY: Mouton Publishers, 1973.

Jung, Carl G. *Man And His Symbols*. New York: Doubleday Publishing Company, 1969.

Karohs, Erika Margarete. *The Analysts' Handbook*. San Francisco: Z-Graphic Publications, 1983.

The Good vs. The Bad Credit Risk As Seen Through Handwriting. San Francisco: Z-Graphic Publications, 1983.

Kellogg, Rhoda. *Analyzing Children's Art*. Palo Alto, CA: Mayfield Publishing Co., 1970.

What Children Scribble And Why. Palo Alto, CA: N. P. Publications, 1955.

King, Leslie, and Christina S. Petersen. *Getting Control Of Your Life*. Salt Lake City, UT: Handwriting Consultants International, 1979.

Klages, Ludwig. *Handschrift und Charakter*. Bonn, West Germany: Universitatsbuchhandlung Bouvier GmbH., 1956.

Klein, Felix. *Male And Female In The Handwriting: What Every Graphologist Should Know About The Subject*. San Jose, CA: American Handwriting Analysis Foundation, 1984.

The Psychology Of The Handwriting Of The Child. San Jose, CA: American Handwriting Analysis Foundation, 1984.

Kobut, Heinz. *The Restoration Of The Self*. New York: International Universities Press, Inc., 1977.

Kurtz, Sheila, and Marilyn Lester. *Grapho-Types: A New Slant On Handwriting Analysis*. New York: Crown Publishers, Inc., 1984.

Laird, Donald A., et al. *Psychology: Human Relations & Motivation, 5th edition.* New York: McGraw-Hill Inc., 1975.

Larson, Linda. "Anorexia And Handwriting." *Journal of the Council of Graphological Studies,* Volume VI, #1. July 1983.
Suicide & Self-Destruction. Campbell, CA: Larson Analytical Services, 1984.

Leibel, Charlotte. *Change Your Handwriting, Change Your Life.* Briarcliff Manor, NY: Stein & Day, Publishers, 1972.

La Vialle, Robert F. *Thirty-Six Illustrated Handwriting Traits For The Supervisor And Manager.* Ardmore, PA: Dorrance & Company, Inc., 1978.

Lester, David. *The Psychological Basis Of Handwriting Analysis: The Relationship Of Handwriting To Personality & Psychopathology.* Chicago: Nelson-Hall Publishers, 1981.

Levinson, Thea St. "Dynamic Disturbances In The Handwriting Of Psychotics." *American Journal of Psychiatry,* Volume 97, #1. 1940.

Lewinson, T. S., and J. Zubin. *Handwriting Analysis: A Series Of Scales For Evaluating The Dynamics Aspects Of Handwriting.* New York: Kings Crown Press (Columbia University Press), 1942.

Link, Betty K. *Graphology: A Tool For Personnel Selection.* Minneapolis, MN: Paul S. Amidon & Associates, Inc., 1983.

Lucas, DeWitt B. *Handwriting & Character Analysis.* Bridgeport, CT: Associated Booksellers, 1959.

McLaughlin, Beverlee S. *Clearer Mirror On My Wall.* Santana, CA: Gallagher Publications, 1980.

McMenamin, Barbera, and Marilyn Martin. *Right Writing.* Spring Valley, CA: Cursive Writing Associates, 1980.

Mann, Peggy. *The Telltale Line: The Secrets Of Handwriting Analysis.* New York: Macmillan Publishing Company, 1976.

Marcuse, Irene. *Guide To The Disturbed Personality Through Handwriting.* New York: Arco Publishing Co., Inc., 1969.

Marley, John. *Handwriting Analysis Made Easy.* North Hollywood, CA: Wilshire Book Company, 1983.

Marne, Patricia. *Crime & Sex In Handwriting.* Piscataway, NJ: New Century Education Corp., 1982.

Mendel, Alfred O. *Personality In Handwriting: A Handbook Of American Graphology, 2nd edition.* New York: Frederick Ungar Publishing Co., Inc., 1981.

Metzler, Mary. *Letters Of The Alphabet Analyzed*. Oakdale, PA: Analytical Handwriting Experts, 1984.

   Scribbles: How To Anaylze Them. Oakdale, PA: Analytical Handwriting Experts, 1981.

Meyer, Jerome S. *The Handwriting Analyzer*. New York: Simon & Schuster, Inc., 1974.

Miller, James. *Bibliography Of Handwriting Analysis: A Graphological Index*. Troy, NY: Whitson Publishing Company, Inc., 1983.

   Handwriting Analysis—A Symbolic Approach. Troy, NY: Whitson Publishing Company, Inc., 1983.

Moretti, Girolamo M., O.F.M. *The Saints Through Their Handwriting*. New York: Macmillan Publishing Company, 1964.

Muhl, A. M. "Handwriting As A Diagnostic Aid." *Journal of the New York Medical Association*, Volume 5, pps. 312-315, 1950.

Myer, Oscar N. *The Language Of Handwriting: And How To Read It*. New York: Frederick Ungar Publishing Co., Inc., 1983.

Olyanova, Nadya. *Handwriting Tells*. North Hollywood, CA: Wilshire Book Company, 1975.

   Psychology Of Handwriting. North Hollywood, CA: Wilshire Book Company, 1960.

Orstein, Robert E. *The Psychology Of Consciousness*. New York: W. H. Freeman & Co., Publishers, 1972.

Overstreet, Bonaro W. *Understanding Fear*. New York: Harper & Row, Publishers, Inc., 1951.

Pelton, Robert W. *Handwriting And Drawings Reveal Your Child's Personality*. New York: Hawthorn Books, Inc., 1973.

Preyor, William T. *Relating To The Psychology Of Handwriting, 2nd edition*. Leipzig, Germany: L. Voss, 1928.

Robie, Joan H. *What Your Handwriting Tells About You*. Nashville, TN: Broadman Press, 1978.

Rockwell, Frances. *Graphology For Lovers*. New York: The New American Library, Inc., 1979.

Roman, Klara G. *Encyclopedia Of The Written Word: A Lexicon For Graphology And Other Aspects Of Writing*. New York: Frederick Ungar Publishing Co., Inc., 1968.

   Handwriting: A Key To Personality. New York: Pantheon Books, Inc., 1977.

Rosen, Billie. *The Science Of Handwriting Analysis*. New York: Bonanza Books, 1965.

Rubin, A., and H. Blair. "The Effects Of Alcohol On Handwriting". *Journal of Clinical Psychology*, Volume 91, pps. 184-287, 1953.

Ruch, Floyd L. *Psychology And Life, 8th edition*. Glenview, IL: Scott, Foresman & Co., 1983.

Ruiz, Mary, and Karen S. Amend. *The Complete Book Of Handwriting Analysis*. North Hollywood, CA: Newcastle Publishing Co., Inc., 1980.

Saudek, Robert. *Anonymous Letters: A Study In Crime And Handwriting*. New York: A. M. S. Press, 1976.

Experiments With Handwriting. Sacramento, CA: Books For Professionals, 1978.

The Psychology Of Handwriting. Sacramento, CA: Books For Professionals, 1978.

Schindler, John. *How To Live Three Hundred And Sixty-Five Days A Year*. New York: Ballantine/Del Rey/Fawcett Books, 1978.

Schweighofer, Fritz. *Graphology & Psychoanalysis: The Handwriting Of Sigmund Freud & His Circle*. New York: Springer Publishing Co., Inc., 1979.

Silver, James F., and Margaret Moyer. *Script Metrics*. Mt. Holly, NJ: Script Metrics, 1983.

Silvi, John. *Handwriting And The Human Mind*. Detroit, MI: Harlo Press, 1973.

Simpson, Diane. *Graphology*. Wakefield, England: E P Publishing Ltd., 1982.

Singer, Eric. *Manual of Graphology, 2nd edition*. London: Gerald Duckworth & Co., Ltd., 1974.

Personality In Handwriting, 2nd edition. London: Gerald Duckworth & Co., Ltd., 1974.

Solomon, Shirl. *How To Really Know Yourself Through Your Handwriting*. New York: Taplinger Publishing Co., Inc., 1973.

Knowing Your Child Through His Handwriting & Drawings. New York: Berkley Publishing Group/Ace Books, 1982.

Sonneman, Ulrich. *Handwriting Analysis*. New York: Grune & Stratton, Inc., 1964.

Sovik, Nils. *Developmental Cybernetics Of Handwriting & Graphic Behavior*. New York: Columbia University Press, 1975.

Stoller, Richard J. *Why Johnny Burns His Schools Down*. New York: Vantage Press, Inc., 1978.

Teltscher, Herry O. *Handwriting—Revelation Of Self*. New York: Hawthorn Books, Inc., 1971.

Thewlis, Malford W., and Isabelle C. Swezy. *Handwriting And The Emotions.* New York: American Graphological Society, 1954.

Thompson, Charlotte Kiser. *Correlation Of Adlerian Psychology And Graphology.* San Jose, CA: American Handwriting Analysis Foundation, 1984.

West, Peter. *Graphology: Understanding What Handwriting Reveals.* York Beach, ME: Samuel Weiser, Inc., 1981.

Westergaard, Marjorie. *Directory Of Handwriting Analysts, 7th edition.* Warren, MI: Marjorie Westergaard, 1985.

Whiting, Eldene C. G. *Glossary Of Standard Terms Used In Handwriting Analysis.* San Diego, CA: Handwriting Consultants of San Diego, 1984.

Printing: The Graphologist's Enigma. San Diego, CA: Handwriting Consultants of San Diego, 1983.

Why Graphologists Should Study The Homosexual Personality. Santee, CA: Graphology Consultants, 1984.

Whiting, Eldene, and Peter Blazi. *Trait Match: Discovering The Occupational Personality Through Handwriting Analysis.* Seattle, WA: Vulcan Books Publishing Co., 1977.

Whiting, Eldene, and Jean Lowerison. *Honesty.* San Jose, CA: American Handwriting Analysis Foundation, 1984.

Williamson, Doris M., and Antoinette E. Meenach. *Cross-Check System for Forgery and Question Document Examination.* Chicago: Nelson-Hall Publishers, 1981.

Wolff, Werner. *Diagrams Of The Unconscious: Handwriting & Personality In Measurement, Experiment & Analysis.* New York: Grune & Stratton, Inc., 1965.

Wyland, Johanna L. *Your Paths In Ink: Graphoanalysis & The Personality.* Smithtown, NY: Exposition Press, Inc., 1980.

Zmuda, Joseph. *Automatic Writing: A Way To The Unconscious Mind.* San Francisco: Z-Graphic Publications, 1983.

Index